'*The Yoga Teacher's Survival Guide* shines in its capacity to engage in critical thinking and question the established norms within the yoga profession. The authors' dedication to scrutinizing these issues is admirable, prompting readers to re-evaluate their own perceptions and practices. The book's critique serves as a stark reminder that no field is without its flaws, and it compels us to address these shortcomings for the betterment of yoga as a whole.'

    – Amy Wheeler, PhD, Former Board President of the International Association of Yoga Therapists (2018–2020)

'Exhausted by daily engagement with the web of contradictions woven around post-modern yoga? Lost in the abysmal crack between the wellness industry and authentic yoga teaching? Alienated by the beach-and-bikini yoga lifestyle portrayed on social media? Then this is the book for you!'

    – Jess Glenny, Elder Yoga Teacher, Registered Yoga Therapist, writer

'Incisive, revealing, uncompromising, and poignant. A much-needed factual and personal spotlight on the reality of teaching modern yoga.'

    – John Stirk, author of *The Original Body: Primal Movement for Yoga Teachers* and *Deeper Still: Authentic Embodiment for Yoga Teachers*

'An outstanding practical intervention that directly explores the painful paradoxes of teaching yoga. This book offers valuable questions, wise reflections, and suggestions based on personal experience. Above all, it offers hope. It is grounded in, but not stifled by, the latest academic research on yoga.'

    – Suzanne Newcombe, author of *Yoga in Britain: Stretching Spirituality and Educating Yogis* and co-editor with Karen O'Brien-Kop of the *Routledge Handbook of Yoga and Meditation Studies*

The Yoga Teacher's Survival Guide

THE YOGA TEACHER'S SURVIVAL GUIDE

Social Justice, Science,
Politics, and Power

Edited by
Theo Wildcroft
and Harriet McAtee

Foreword by Matthew Remski

SINGING DRAGON
LONDON AND PHILADELPHIA

First published in Great Britain in 2024 by Singing Dragon,
an imprint of Jessica Kingsley Publishers
Part of John Murray Press

1

Content Warning: This book mentions abuse and trauma.

A CIP catalogue record for this title is available from the
British Library and the Library of Congress

ISBN 978 1 80501 166 8
eISBN 978 1 80501 167 5

Printed and bound in Great Britain by CPI Group (UK)

Jessica Kingsley Publishers' policy is to use papers that are natural, renewable and recyclable
products and made from wood grown in sustainable forests. The logging and manufacturing
processes are expected to conform to the environmental regulations of the country of origin.

Singing Dragon
Carmelite House
50 Victoria Embankment
London EC4Y 0DZ

www.singingdragon.com

John Murray Press
Part of Hodder & Stoughton Limited
An Hachette UK Company

Contents

Teaching, Agency, and Trauma

Race. Justice. Equity.

Money and Power

Foreword

This *Survival Guide* will arrive in print only a few years – or months – before a Silicon Valley tech bro who went to a few hot yoga classes in 2018 hoovers every yoga video, Insta reel, and 'Yoga means Union' blog post into a startup AI blender. He'll let it churn, then type in a few prompts, and a constellation of yoga teacher avatars will spawn like neo-Tantric deities on a holodeck.

The user will choose a body skin, athleisure print, exotic practice venue, yoga style and century, class theme, charisma quotient, and an intensity level on a scale from 'somatic dominance' to 'trauma informed'. A Woo Slider can set a preference of pseudoscientific versus evidence-based objectives.

For a per-use fee, the yoga app will demonstrate poses in perfect 4K while reciting a curated mix of all the cues the AI scraped, from Iyengar to Bizzie Gold of Buti Yoga. She can have the voice of Cardi B or Brené Brown. In later iterations – according to customer demand – the AI may even allow the user to filter out antivax slogans and QAnon dogwhistles.

This new absurdity will not surprise the writers in this volume. It's just another existential challenge to a spiritual subculture perennially seeking a reality principle and a community ethos.

Gathered here are folks who survived the yoga cults of the 1980s. They weathered the growth bubble of the 1990s and the aughts, and saw that their new 'industry' was complicit in the cruelty of gentrification. They were harassed and marginalized and offered Lululemon Ambassadorships for their troubles. They suffered repetitive stress injuries due to a complete lack of biomechanics education. They've watched essential oil MLMs (multi-level marketing schemes) cannibalize entire communities because the side hustle of yoga teaching needs a side hustle to work. They've watched an old-but-new heteronormative orthodoxy emerge through the marketing of 'divine feminine' and 'divine masculine' workshops. They knew that many of their colleagues were just one more juice fast away from going all-in on body fascism and soft eugenics.

In the 2010s, many of the writers in this volume began to agitate in fringe but impassioned campaigns for accessibility, higher education standards, more stringent ethics, postcolonial awareness, abuse accountability, and labor justice. They rallied against ableism, orientalism, and the lie that self-care could substitute for robust health policy.

Things were hard, but looking up. In 2019, yoga teachers in New York State met with labor leaders to start unionization talks, and voted to go forward. The yoga #MeToo wave crested that same year, prompting exposés and lawsuits. When it was clear that the leaders of Sivananda Yoga were not going to fully investigate documented intergenerational abuse in their own organization, survivors and allies organized, crowdfunded, and published their own investigation. It was incredible.

Then, all of these efforts ground to a halt in the spring of 2020, when COVID shuttered yoga spaces, bankrupted several large yoga companies, disrupted yoga Facebook with fever dreams, and handed online yoga streamers a license to print money, and to open a fresh gateway between yoga and reactionary politics. That's not an exaggeration, as I can relate through a funny-not-funny story involving several of the people in this book.

When Davy Jones of the Brighton Yoga Festival was working to organize a panel featuring survivors of institutional abuse in yoga in 2019, I helped broker a deal with Yoga International (YI) where they would shoulder break-even expenses in exchange for professional video documentation of the event, and rights to host it – on the condition it would never be paywalled. I had a hunch the deal would work because at that time the platform was run by GenZ progressives who were also platforming decolonizing, anti-ableist, and evidence-based content.

The groundbreaking event, moderated by Theo Wildcroft, won broad acclaim on the Yoga International platform. But at the end of 2021, to the shock of everyone who worked there, YI was gobbled up by the largest conspiracy theory and pseudoscience platform in the world, GaiaTV. With close to 700,000 paying subscribers at $11.99 a month, Gaia brings in over $107 million a year in revenue. Acquiring Yoga International bought another 300,000 subscribers, who would have been paying either $9.99 a month or $99 for the year. But more than the money, GaiaTV nabbed a diverse content archive that elevated and laundered their brand. Suddenly, the panel discussion, and the work of people like Jivana Heyman disappeared behind a paywall, where it sat beside seminars by the reptilian illuminati believer David Icke and Pretendian shamans who claim to speak to angels.

Luckily, Jones got GaiaTV to surrender the content with a few stern Green-Party-style letters. But the sequence of events reads like an elevator pitch for a season of 'Yoga at the Crossroad'. After decades of silence, survivors of sexual assault in high-demand yoga groups are finally given a platform at the most progressive festival in the world, supported by exemplary scholars and advocates. Their stories are briefly promoted by a legit company, but as the chaos of COVID peaks, they are bought and monetized by the Netflix of New Age bullshit. And then they took those stories back, and carried on.

The writers in this volume know very well that globalization, commodification, and technologization over the past century have transformed mainstream yoga into the religion of the neoliberal order, while promising women empowerment and gig workers freedom, and funneling the money to the top. They know that the AI tech bro isn't that different from the Boomer yoga tycoon who was always more about sales than substance, who plagiarized and recycled their content to feed their lucrative downlines. They know that the yoga discourse that will always pay the highest will be the discourse that enhances magical thinking, spiritual bypassing, and various flavors of orientalism. They know that a neoliberal religion is meant to consecrate the status quo, to bless the endless social reproduction of ideal bodies, purity fetishes, and productivity hacks. They have seen how easy it was for capitalism to sell yoga as a method for reinforcing rather than breaking our conditioning.

How do they know these things? Because they brought feminism, queerness, anti-ableism, anti-racism, and dog-eared copies of *Pedagogy of the Oppressed* with them. Because among them are abuse survivors, social workers, AIDS activists, anti-racist facilitators, labor organizers, and the neurodiverse. Because they remembered that Rosa Parks practiced yoga. In this book, they've laid it all out on the line.

They remembered their roots, their origins, even as the captains of the yoga industry tried to sell them magic beans and a saffronized enlightenment. In cult recovery theory, we often speak about the long, slow repair of the 'pre-cult self' – that part of you that remained impervious to indoctrination. The essential thing is to realize it can always be reawakened by friends. That's what I think this book is. A kind of gentle alarm clock, rousing you, again, not to the grind that the tech bro is waiting to co-opt, but to the core values that have always provoked your reverie, love, and action.

If you can eat, pay rent, support your dependents, and afford health care, there is one thing to say about being a visionary in a precarious discipline that does not know what it is, in an economy that doesn't want to pay you, in a world longing for meaning. It can turn you into an expert in creating that 'third space' that capitalism always tries to pinch off. This is the space that all the radical urban planners are now talking about. It's neither where you sleep nor where you work. The space where you can change your conditioning and your local culture with the shared activities no AI can mimic. Where you can decide how best to apply your love and your skill in the face of rising fascism and temperatures.

This book is also a third space, where you may learn that you could go on teaching yoga, or you could organize a community garden, and it's all the same. Both are more offline than on. And in both places you will have told the bullies, 'You're not in charge anymore. We're making a better place. We don't know what it will look like. But you can lend a hand if you want.'

Matthew Remski

Author of *Practice and All Is Coming: Abuse, Cult Dynamics, and Healing in Yoga and Beyond* (2019); co-author of *Conspirituality: How New Age Conspiracy Theories Became a Health Threat*

Acknowledgements

Harriet and Theo would like to thank all the contributors to this book for their generosity and care in responding to our invitation. Behind them is a wide and disparate network of other wise people we could have also asked to write chapters for this book, as well as every student, trainee, colleague, and researcher in the communities of practice that support us. It continues to be a privilege to share with you all both the practice of yoga and the conversations it provokes. May this book be everything you deserve and more.

We'd also like to thank the team who turned this manuscript into something you can hold in your hands, including our publishers, as well as those unsung heroes who taught us not just to write, but to edit, which is a far more useful skill.

Like all writers, for us, there are also those people whose presence in one's daily life makes all this possible. For Theo that is Phil (for full-time love and logistics), but also Carrie (for invaluable part-time organization), and definitely Storm the greyhound (for good vibes as always). For Harriet that is Erwan (*merci mon cœur*), her wonderful team at Nourish (especially assistant-extraordinaire, Katie) and the fur babies (Pickles and Loki).

INTRODUCTION

'HAVE YOU TRIED YOGA?'

If you read the question in our title for this introduction and sighed and rolled your eyes, then this is probably the yoga book for you. When we, Harriet, and Theo, read those words, we just feel very tired. But then, all the yoga teachers we know are very tired most of the time.

In the saturated market of yoga and wellness, it might be useful for us to begin by telling you what sort of yoga book this is not. This is not a comprehensive textbook. We are not offering you a firm and final say on what is right and what is wrong. There are no protocols", no prescriptions, no lists of contraindications or recommendations. We won't be talking about how to practise or teach *trikonāsana* (or any other pose). There are no photographs of models performing *āsana*s with perfectly coiffed hair or perfectly positioned props. There are no checklists, no anatomical explanations, no sequencing suggestions.

At this point, you might be wondering what you've spent your hard-earned money on, and for yoga teachers, we know that money is both hard-earned and never substantive enough. This is a book born from the recognition that the friends, colleagues, elders, and students around us were facing real crises in their yoga teaching, and struggling to live well through teaching yoga, whether on a financial, emotional, physical, or spiritual level. We wanted to write a book which spoke to those who might be feeling disillusioned, lost, lonely, or despairing at the state of contemporary yoga. We wanted to offer respite from shallow solutions and the co-opting of serious systemic issues for authority and credibility.

There are so many books that promise to deliver the one universal truth about yoga teaching, and the existence of such books does suggest that there is a hunger for simple and accessible answers. Yoga teachers are uncertain: about their place in capitalism, about their contribution to health, about their relationship to ancient and long-maligned cultures and to social justice and international politics. Sometimes we are even uncertain about whether we are good people and whether there's a point to what we're doing.

So we – Harriet and Theo – took a step back and decided to take a wider view of the biggest questions that are troubling yoga teachers today. We have synthesized the most common worries of yoga teachers in our trainings into the six themes of this book: critical thinking; honouring our sources; scientific enquiries; trauma; race and equity; and finally money and power. We approached some of the yoga teachers we most respect, offered them a theme, and asked them to write what they think yoga teachers most need to hear. They started from simple questions: What can we know about the history of yoga? Is stretching really good for you? How do we reconcile money with a spiritual practice? How can we practise honourably together, given the enduring effects of colonialism and racism?

Contemplating each of these simple questions provokes a particular crisis: a shedding of preconceptions and assumptions. In the answers, new knowledge is discovered, teaching strategies are found, and personal experience is integrated. The book begins with two such journeys, leading to very different answers. For each subsequent theme, you will find multiple voices, collaborating in mutual respect, and occasionally respectful disagreement. Including those multiple voices was essential. We wanted to bring you more than just our voices. This isn't every scholar and yoga teacher we love and work with, but it is reflective of what Etienne Wenger calls a 'community of practice',[1] and even what bell hooks called a 'beloved community'.[2] It is also a circle of trust in action – all the things that Theo believes are essential to the healthy practice of 'post-lineage yoga'.[3]

But before we get into the details, it is useful to start from common ground.

WHERE WE BEGAN

Before we were yoga teachers and trainers, Theo and Harriet were students and practitioners of yoga. Like many, we found solace, freedom, and comfort through our practice, and felt a desire to deepen practice through training, sharing our experiences and love of yoga with others through teaching.

Fast forward some years, and Theo was sat at a festival with a friend, watching the various practices being shared around her. She gestured furiously, and not for the first time, said, 'Why is no one talking about this?' And her friend replied, 'Theo, either write a book or do a PhD but either way, let me help you.' And that's how her PhD, and her first book (*Post-Lineage Yoga*, 2020) was born.

Meanwhile, kept up at night by the thought of 'shit yoga teachers', Harriet had been driven to create teacher training programmes centred on an inclusive, joyful, person-centred approach. (She cares a lot more about her trainees than this suggests.)

The further we delved into our work and studies as yoga practitioners, teachers, and trainers, the more we encountered similar stories, confessions, and cathartic sharings from fellow students and teachers. Whether it was a teacher sharing a challenging or dangerous encounter with a student, or a trainee sharing concerns about their experiences with a previous teacher training, or a student sense-checking the latest outlandish claim from their previously trusted yoga teacher, sometimes it felt that at every turn we were confronted by yet another story which made us roll our eyes or shake our heads, or broke our hearts a little.

Most yoga teachers, we are sure, do not set out to do harm. The intention for most as they embark on their training and teaching journeys is to share the practices that have brought them ease and empowerment with others. This is an admirable and common intention, and one that should be celebrated. It is our hope that this book helps to support yoga teachers in this endeavour, by offering ways to think critically about what 'everyone knows' about yoga, by unpacking the ways in which some of the aspects of contemporary yoga reinforces harmful dynamics and systems of oppression, and by posing constructive questions about what it means to practise and teach yoga today.

WHAT 'EVERYONE KNOWS' ABOUT YOGA

Millions of practitioners around the world currently engage in a multitude of practices that they all call 'yoga'. This term covers a vast diversity and rich history of practice, philosophy, and belief. But today, the mainstream image of yoga is of bodies moving and bodies sitting for general health and wellbeing. This is what academics most often call 'modern postural yoga', after the groundbreaking research of Elizabeth De Michelis,[4] or sometimes 'post-lineage yoga'.[5]

Visions of slender, female flexibility and privileged calm dominate the marketing of some extremely profitable international industries.[6] A quick search of global media sources reveals some staggering statistics, but far fewer concrete sources for those statistics.

The website MedAlertHelp reports that there are more than 300 million yoga practitioners around the world, and the global yoga industry generated $37.46 billion in 2019.[7] Zippia projects this figure to grow to $66.23 billion by 2027.[8] Statista.com declared the US market to have generated $9.31 billion alone in 2020.[9] Finder UK claimed a UK revenue for 'the Pilates and yoga industry' of over £926 million in 2020, with up to 460,000 UK residents taking part in yoga classes every week.[10] And most confidently of all, Comparecamp claims the current global yoga industry to be worth more than $84 billion.[11]

Yet the data for these claims are unclear. Park, Braun, and Siegel conducted one comparative research study to discover: what do we know about who practises yoga? They complained that:

> Most research on yoga has focused on determining its effects, often relying on experimental designs or clinical trials. Other studies have relied on case reports or surveys of convenience samples to compare those who do versus those who do not use yoga on some outcome measure. While important for understanding the effects of yoga on health and well-being, these studies do not provide information on a more general question: who does yoga?[12]

Such studies often fail to give any detail of the content of the practice being studied.

Alternatively, we can discover through a YouTube search that the most popular yoga-tagged channel, *Yoga with Adriene*, has 11.2 million subscribers as of July 2022,[13] and we can at least know exactly what Adriene considers to be a sensible yoga practice. But we cannot measure active or regular participation, only how many people have glanced at a video.

Occasionally, polling organizations are commissioned by the yoga industry itself to ask a few questions. A landmark 2016 study by IPSOS for Yoga Alliance, for example, found that yoga practitioners' *self-reported* spending on yoga classes and equipment was equivalent, multiplied to a national scale, to over $16 million.[14] But that figure is little more than an educated guess. A more recent study by the UK Yoga Teachers Union reported on the working landscape of yoga teaching. Again, a self-selected population was asked for self-reported data on how often they teach, how much they earn, and so on.[15]

There is little truly reliable global or national data about how many people practise 'yoga', what they even mean when they use the term, and how the practice relates to the economy. Commonly shared statistics on the benefits of, the earnings of, and participation in contemporary yoga are not as robust as they first appear.

The very prevalence of yoga 'statistics', media comment pieces, and exploratory medical studies demonstrates that from health to tourism, and business to education, interest in 'yoga' is a globally important phenomenon.

But there seems to be much less mainstream interest in defining yoga, as a historical practice, as an adjunct medical intervention, or as a global wellbeing phenomenon.

Yoga teachers, as a whole, are much more invested in discovering the answers to those questions. For most people, yoga is one of those things that 'everyone knows' about. And yet what 'everyone knows' is that yoga is ancient and modern, religious and secular. It makes you fit, and aids relaxation. It is commercial and traditional. It is both Indian and transnational.

The differences in form and intention between different forms of yoga as historical practice, yoga as health intervention, and yoga as marketing meme can be glaring.[16] And as most yoga teachers know, unpicking the diversity of yoga inevitably entangles us in debates about nationalism and appropriation, racism and colonialism, neo-liberalism, self-surveillance, and eugenics. Yoga has shaped nations, cultures, and communities, and has been shaped by them in turn. Heated debates about the 'authenticity' of specific practice forms, the extraction of wisdom techniques for commercial gain, and the 'true' meaning of the practice dominate contemporary transnational yoga discourse.

YOGA TEACHING AND YOGA RESEARCH

To generalize, there is a yoga 'industry' that promotes yoga as a benign, health-forwarding practice, supported by ill-defined ancient and spiritual roots, allied to modern technologies and pedagogical techniques, which supports an ever-growing profit base to the benefit of all nations. Rather less visible in the cultural mainstream is the diverse global collective of yoga teachers and long-term practitioners who understand that practices considered to be 'traditional' are in many cases a modern invention, that the science of yoga is at best unproven, that you can indeed be injured in a yoga class, and that there is no specific posture that will cure your lower back pain.

That teaching collective is also variously, but increasingly, aware that sexual abuse, toxic working practices, and all manner of ethical transgressions are endemic within the yoga 'industry' worldwide. In that, yoga teachers are not unique, but perhaps uniquely placed to suffer, given the gendered and precarious nature of the work and the holistic, even all-encompassing nature of the practice. Yoga teaching may be a safe working environment for some and a reliable income source for few, but is a spiritual identity for many.

The teaching of yoga is largely unregulated. Yoga teachers are struggling to professionalize and organize, to their own benefit and solidarity, but also in response to demands for exactly the safe and predictable, health-forwarding adjunct health intervention that educational and health organizations have been promised.

Perhaps most interestingly, as a result, yoga teaching as a profession benefits from an extremely close relationship to research into yoga as a practice. Internationally, an MA in yoga studies from SOAS (the School of Oriental and African Studies at London University) in the UK, LMU (Loyola Marymount University) in the US, or a small number of other providers can function as an unofficial 'advanced' qualification for yoga education providers. Scholars of yoga are contracted to provide content for accessible independent platforms such as Yogic Studies and SOAS' Centre of Yoga Studies, as well as dropping into guest teach on yoga teacher training programmes.

Scholar–practitioner relationships can be complex at best in this small but steadily growing field of study. Research into yoga can be eagerly awaited, or vehemently rejected by yoga communities. The impact of Mark Singleton's *Yoga Body* (2010), James Mallinson and Mark Singleton's *Roots of Yoga* (2017), and similar texts is just one reason why we are starting to see the persistent myth of 'traditional yoga' as a singular, coherent, and unchanging practice come to an end, but it is also why at least some yoga studies researchers avoid social media entirely.[17]

Together, academic researchers and teacher-practitioners (and those that are both) are discovering that both the roots and present reality of yoga practice are diverse, fragmented, and heavily blended, and intentions and effects for practitioners are equally diverse, complex, and contingent on circumstance. Even yoga scholars have noticed that there is a 'hunger in the yoga community for writing about yoga that is critical, challenging, political, and relevant to life in the 21st century'.[18]

NAVIGATING THIS BOOK

Our collection begins, therefore, with 'Thinking Critically'. In Chapter 1, 'I Am Not a Teacher Any Longer', Karin Carlson sets out the differences between practising yoga and teaching yoga, and between yoga and the yoga industry. Her critical evaluation of what it means and what it takes to teach yoga today suggests, provocatively, that professionalization might actually erode what is life-affirming about our practice.

In contrast, Donna Farhi's chapter, 'Falling Short of Knowing' (Chapter 2), maintains the same ambivalence to teaching yoga as an industry, but offers the hope that we might be able to create a space of sanctuary, holding back both commercial imperatives and therapeutic expectations long enough for students and teachers to relate more authentically through yoga.

The themes that these two pieces share – ambivalence to the institutionalization of yoga, personal evolution, living with unknowing, and the centrality of relationships to teaching – recur time and again throughout this collection.

Our next section is 'Honouring Our Sources', and speaks to one of the most common issues for yoga teachers: how to accurately reflect and respect the pre-modern roots of our contemporary practices in our teaching. Chapter 3, 'History – a Dialogue, a Commentary, and Footnotes', co-written by Barbora Sojková, Simran Uppal, and Theo and Harriet ourselves, encourages the reader to ask: what can we know about the history of yoga?

In Chapter 4, 'Tools for Teaching Non-Dogmatic Yoga History', Barbora Sojková returns. She sets out simple teaching and citation practices, shares her key takeaways for the history of yoga, and adds a wonderful primer of resources to guide further reading.

Finally for this section, Simran Uppal contributes Chapter 5, 'Six Verses on Becoming Tulsidas', a personal reflection on what 'honouring our sources' means in the context of being a queer, South Asian, diasporic yoga teacher and practitioner. Taken together, this section provides the conceptual framework, the practical tools, the further resources, and the inspiration to equip yoga teachers with confidence in tackling this perennial issue.

Our third section is 'Scientific Enquiries into Yoga'. Throughout its modern history, yoga has had an ambivalent relationship to science. On the one hand, new scientific theories pass through yoga culture like a meme or a contagious force. On the other hand, practitioners are often drawn to alternative systems of knowledge, treating scientific research as a cumbersome beast, struggling to verify what practitioners, or alternative therapists, or traditional medicines 'already know'.

We begin with Jules Mitchell's chapter, 'The Science of Yoga Re-Examined' (Chapter 6), inviting you to reflect on the relationship between function, performance, and injury in yoga practice. Along the way, we gain a flavour of Jules' own fascinating journey through the scientific research process.

Peter Blackaby's chapter, 'Enquiry and Intention in the Teaching of Yoga' (Chapter 7), explores the relationship between intention and attention, using this to differentiate between exercise, performance, and yoga, and encouraging us to understand the unique place that yoga holds as a mode of bodily enquiry. Like Peter, we believe a somatic approach is one of the most effective ways to integrate contemporary scientific understandings into a traditional yogic approach of self-discovery and self-awareness.

Finally in this section, Beverley Nolan offers a chapter called 'Head, Heart, and Hands' (Chapter 8). It is a deep and at times vulnerable meditation on the role of the teacher in facilitating learning about anatomy through experience, while at the same time challenging hierarchies and supporting the discovery of each student's unique inner teacher.

More and more yoga teachers are ready to discuss the patterns of behaviour and structures of power that enable abusers to take advantage of the yoga teacher–student relationship. We have also seen a rise in the use of yoga in therapeutic settings, where students have pre-existing conditions, might have suffered adverse events, and may be vulnerable in diverse ways. It is no surprise, then, that there is a common conversation happening about how to make yoga 'safe' for those suffering the effects of trauma, as well as how to make yoga spaces 'safe' from abuse.

Sadly, absolute safety is impossible, but in examining the tangled issues of student agency, safety, and trauma, we can learn a lot about more effective, appropriate, and ethical teaching strategies. Thus our next section is 'Teaching, Agency, and Trauma'. For obvious reasons, the whole section comes with a 'strong content' note for mentions of trauma, abuse, suffering, and suicide.

To begin, Amelia Wood's chapter, 'Trauma, Yoga, and Spiritual Abuse' (Chapter 9), offers a history of 'trauma-informed care'. It considers the politics of trauma-informed approaches and the structural nature of trauma, and reminds us that marginalized groups are both more likely to suffer trauma and less able to access spaces to heal. Like Amelia, we believe that yoga teaching always holds the potential to both harm and heal, and that improving student agency is the key to the latter.

Chapter 10, 'Person-Centred Teaching for Trauma', is a guide to the main principles that can make yoga teaching more sensitive to the experiences of trauma. Harriet and Laura Wilson demonstrate how to facilitate student-centred experiences of empowerment and agency, and include a set of enquiries for those interested in pursuing further training.

We, Harriet and Theo, are both survivors of long-term, interpersonal abuse. We know that conversations about trauma between survivors are very different to conversations with non-survivors. There is a common ground, not of experience, but of tone: a familiarity with dark humour and complex emotions, an understanding that the world is home to both more pain and more joy than many people realize. With Chapter 11, 'On Surviving', then, we include a conversation exploring such themes as: being a 'good survivor' and the fatigue of survivorship, the fallacy of 'completion' in healing, the dangers of prioritizing the practice over the person, and the reality of being both broken and healed at the same time.

Yoga's history in the service of empire and independence, colonialism and nationalism, is long and complex. The next section, 'Race. Justice. Equity.' was essential to include in this book. As white, working-class women who have benefited from colonial histories, Harriet and Theo are immensely grateful for the solidarity of friends, collaborators, and co-conspirators who are people of colour in so many aspects of our work. This book is no exception.

Sheena Sood's 'Introducing Omwashing' (Chapter 12) delivers a much-needed reframing of yoga and cultural appropriation, through the lens of orientalism. This chapter contains a vital critique of the current mainstream solutions, which all too often reinforce racial capitalism, caste-based oppression, and far-right ethno-nationalism.

In Chapter 13, 'Anti-Racist Pedagogy as an Act of Love', Simran Uppal brings us a radically anti-racist pedagogy. Like Sheena, Simran critiques the appropriation of representation politics by corporate equality and diversity initiatives, but this is a more practical chapter, which moves beyond theory as well as beyond the tick-box exercises and performative white guilt of many courses in racial 'awareness'.

Finally for this section, Aisha Nash's 'Breathing Out Loud' (Chapter 14) describes the violence that is done through our racialized assumptions about what a 'healthy' body looks and feels like. Aisha shows us how the intersection of yoga and race can be used in the service of either appropriative harm or reclaimed healing, unpeeling the layers of hypocrisy and violence in the wellness industry, and the grief, rage, and empowerment that results.

Our final section is 'Money and Power'. Navigating an ambivalent relationship to commerce and industry is an ever-present reality for yoga teachers. But financial relationships and inequities also reflect and reinforce other forms of interpersonal and societal power. Without a strong foundational understanding of how money and power flow through yoga teaching, we are always vulnerable to exploitation.

In Chapter 15, 'Yoga Means Union', Laura Hancock draws on her work with the UK's first yoga teaching trades union to deliver a clear-sighted and uncompromising examination of burnout, precarity, bullying, and sexual harassment within yoga teaching as an industry.

If Laura's chapter is a much-needed, sober account of money and power in yoga teaching, both Chapter 16 by Davy Jones and Chapter 17 by Jivana Heyman are potential messages of hope. In 'Brighton Yoga Festival', Davy is clear about the disconnect between yoga teaching at the grassroots level and yoga as a commercial industry. This is a glimpse into a life of hard work and uneasy compromises, of authentic relationships, and of leveraging privilege to a greater good.

Finally, with 'Jivana's Homework', Jivana Heyman offers a more personal reflection on using some of the teachings of yoga philosophy to frame our interactions with money and power. Most of all, this chapter demonstrates how opening yourself up to the relationship between money and power in yoga leaves you with more questions than answers. His conclusion, and ours, is that leaning into these questions with an attitude of openness, non-attachment, service, and community is the only way for change to happen.

INTEGRATING THIS BOOK

We feel it's important to include a brief list of suggestions and thoughts on how to engage with and integrate this book, largely because the content covered is at points both vast and personal, both universal and intimate. That requires a sense of care for ourselves and time to process, but we also hope this book will be something you want to return to, to re-read and revisit over time.

First, we encourage you to begin with whatever section most captures your imagination. Begin with the subject that most strikes a chord in your heart. The pieces in this book speak to each other in a non-linear way: themes repeat and circle back on themselves, revealing more interconnections and questions each time. That being said, the book also works perfectly well if you start at the start and end at the end.

Second, we encourage you to take your time. The ideas discussed are often beautiful and inspirational, but also sometimes provocative and challenging. One of the biggest injuries capitalism and white supremacy have done to our culture is insinuating a sense of urgency deep inside many of us: a feeling that things need to happen today, or tomorrow (or should have happened yesterday). As one of Harriet's favourite resources on white supremacy clarifies, a sense of urgency: '[perpetuates] power [imbalances] while disconnecting us from our need to breathe and pause and reflect. The irony is that this imposed sense of urgency serves to erase the actual urgency of tackling racial and social injustice.'[19] So we encourage you to take your time, allowing space for reflection, connection, and pause. This might look like taking breaks while reading, to stretch your body or wriggle, make your favourite drink, cuddle a pet, water your plants, or stare out of the window. It might also look like allowing pauses to journal, if that's something which works for you, or to make notes. You might find a fellow yoga teacher friend to explore this book together, sharing your reflections, questions, worries, and inspirations. The things you read and the questions they raise might make you feel anything from uncomfortable to angry to amused to motivated. Allow space for yourself to notice what arises, with as much tenderness and as little judgement as possible.

This leads us quite nicely to our third suggestion: we encourage you to allow space for grief, guilt, and anger to arise. Specifically, allow space for grief and even shame, on behalf of past versions of yourself. In 2021, Harriet and her team of regular collaborators (which includes Theo and Simran) set out to significantly revise the training manual for Harriet's 200-hour teacher training programme. At this point, the manual was four years old, and this was the first time major sections of the manual had been completely re-envisioned and rewritten. For Harriet, this provoked a deep sense of grief and an important opportunity to reflect on the growth and development of her teaching philosophy and practice. While this was a moment of appreciation and gratitude, it was also accompanied by a tinge of grief and even guilt.

At the time, Harriet drew strength and resourcing from her collaborators, but also from the ideas of Audre Lorde. In *The Uses of Anger*, Lorde argues for seeing guilt and anger as productive, creative, and empowering:

> Anger is a source of empowerment we must not fear to tap for energy rather than guilt. When we turn from anger we turn from insight, saying we will accept only the designs already known, those deadly and safely familiar. I have tried to learn my anger's usefulness to me, as well as its limitations.[20]

Further, Lorde argues that rather than guilt being a response to anger, 'it is a response to one's own actions or lack of action'.[21] So alongside space to pause, reflect, and grieve, we also encourage you to take time to consider where you might be able to take productive, creative, caring action.

Third, we'd like to introduce you to 'Harriet's Homework' (a riff on 'Jivana's Homework', which you'll encounter in the final piece of this book). In our classes, trainings, and courses, we often find that students put huge pressure on themselves to recall and perfect their attainment of knowledge. Students feel they are a 'good' student or 'good' teacher based on how much they have managed to retain from the training.

In response, Harriet introduced the idea of 'Harriet's Homework': go away and forget everything. Which is another way of saying, do not let your learning get in the way of living your life. Let things marinate and settle. Go to work and love your friends and do the mundane things of everyday life (and maybe some yoga practice), and perhaps just see what comes up, what ideas from this book float to the surface of your mind, demanding to be recalled, discussed, shared.

This book isn't going anywhere, and neither is yoga. There is time and space to read, practise, talk, and live.

Lastly, we encourage you to seek support where needed and wanted. Take good care of yourself, and seek solace where appropriate. This might be talking with friends, mentors, therapists, healthcare providers. Take breaks and take your time.

We decided to embark on this project because it felt needed and deeply necessary. Throughout the writing and editing stages, our working title (originally a joke from Harriet) was 'So You Think You Don't Want to Be a Yoga Teacher Any More?' Hidden beneath this joke are two things: first, a recognition of the real personal and professional crises being experienced by yoga teachers worldwide, and second, the hope that we might be able to offer new approaches (and more questions), to encourage you to continue if you want to, and equally, to offer comfort and acknowledgement if you decide to move on.

Wherever you find yourself in your journey of teaching and practising yoga, we hope this book provides a resource for thinking more deeply about what it means to teach and how. We hope it inspires, uplifts, and empowers, just as much as it might provoke, confuse, and outrage. Let's begin.

THINKING
CRITICALLY

1 ___

I AM NOT A TEACHER ANY LONGER

Karin Carlson

Karin Carlson was, until very recently, a yoga teacher and writer about yoga. Her memoir, *Notes on My Skin*, is currently fishing for a literary agent. Meanwhile Karin is working on a murder mystery novel but hasn't yet figured out who dies. She writes about somatics, semantics, and ethics in her weekly newsletter, *Gristle and Bone*, published through Substack. Karin lives in Minneapolis with the person she loves. She bakes cakes, loves architecture and anatomy, and goes for very long walks almost every single day.

Karin was still a yoga teacher, running an 'Anti-200 hour' course that definitely wasn't a yoga teacher training, when we asked her to write a piece on 'critical thinking for yoga teachers'. What she submitted was so much more than we could have asked for. This piece captures the acute personal and professional crisis that we believe is currently being felt by yoga teachers around the world. With multiple national and international political crises looming, unsure about what yoga teaching will even look like within the next few years, many are abandoning or radically rethinking their teaching careers.

Karin's writing also sets out the differences between practising yoga and teaching yoga, between yoga and the yoga industry. It demonstrates the intimately relational nature of teaching, and the meaninglessness of so much of the industry that surrounds it. This critical evaluation of what it means and what it takes to teach yoga today suggests, provocatively, that professionalization might actually erode what is life-affirming about our practice.

Themes such as ambivalence to the institutionalization of yoga, personal evolution, living with unknowing, and the centrality of relationships to teaching will return in our next chosen piece, but with very different conclusions. Again and again in this collection, you will find mutual respect and common ground leading to diverse answers. This too is yoga, and so we're delighted to begin here.

I've been a yoga teacher for 14 years. I am not a teacher any longer.

This is a recent change. I was teaching and had no intention of quitting when I was asked to write this chapter. I was passionate about the beauty and potential of these practices. I had a deep reverence for the tradition and was openly engaged with the problems of colonialism, capitalism, and abuses of power within the community. I fully believed we could do better.

But that was six months ago.[i] Six months lands differently in this era of social crisis and global pandemic. We sense a tentativeness about our work and our lives, regardless of what industry we're in; the future of our work is unimaginable. Without an imaginable future, time feels like nothing but an accumulation, a detritus of trauma compounding traumas. What was taken as a given opens itself to question; what was right can quickly become untenable. Two months after writing this chapter I announced my resignation from yoga. Having quit, I began to feel squeamish about my contribution to this book.

For me to offer guidance navigating the field felt disingenuous if I was leaving yoga. The yoga industry already struggles with hypocrisy and empty promises. Mewing a little, I asked the editors if they still wanted me to participate. They said yes: maybe leaving the industry says something about the industry. More people leave than stay, and the industry does itself a disservice by not studying that phenomenon.

I have rewritten the piece entirely: I am not now speaking as a mentor of yoga teachers, but as someone who has been there and has decided to leave. I pose teaching as an unanswered question: who says we should teach yoga?

THERE IS A DIFFERENCE BETWEEN YOGA AND THE YOGA INDUSTRY

The universal response to my leaving has been *you mean you're quitting teaching, but not leaving yoga, right?* People say this in lowered voices. They look concerned. A tangle of abandonment and compassion tightens their eyes. My students express grief, my mentors disappointment.

Have I burned out, they wonder. Do I no longer believe? Am I okay?

---

i   Karin was writing this in May 2022.

I am okay. My leaving is not a sad thing. It is the outcome of yoga having done its job. Quitting has more personal integrity to it than soldiering on. I think we have to talk about what we mean when we say yoga, and identify the presumptions we have about its 'practice' and 'teaching'. Like the word 'yoga', the concept 'yoga teacher' is so ambivalent it doesn't mean anything without further context.

I began teaching full time, as my only income, immediately after attending my first training. I never stopped. That simply isn't possible for most folks. I was lucky.

I never wanted to be a yoga teacher. Most people who attend teacher trainings never intend to teach. We went because we were told it was what one does when one becomes a 'serious' yoga student. Some of us were told 'teaching' or 'yoga' was our dharmic path, a kind of hero's journey with all sorts of moralistic implications. I hate when this happens. It implies folks need to buy something if they want to find their souls.

I wasn't ever told this. I got sober and started practising yoga at the same time. In getting sober I'd lost both my home and my job. My yoga advanced in tandem to my life falling apart. I only went to teacher training because it was something to do that didn't involve relapsing.

My life upended. At the time it felt hard, and I felt sorry for myself. I recognize now how blessed I was. My privileges – a family who understood recovery and were able to support me, several years where staying sober and taking care took precedence over making a living wage, a dozen teachers who were more mentor than teacher trainer – allowed me to immerse myself in yoga training and practice like a renunciate. I didn't realize it at the time, but I was closer to traditional study than most contemporary folks: traditionally, yoga teachings were handed on one to one in a mentored way, over the course of a long period of time. I only ever picked up certificates as an afterthought. I taught as a corollary, a side piece, to what I was learning. I spent hours every day with my teachers, picking their brains and getting the equivalent of several private lessons a week. No one gets that in teacher training.

I always knew, because I was experiencing it, that there is a difference between yoga and the yoga industry. Yoga was mysteriously changing who I was. The industry seemed superfluous.

The real kicker is I was good at it. Teaching, I mean. Not that I am a particularly 'good' yoga teacher. I mean the best things I've ever done in my life I've done in my role as yoga teacher.

I'd never been good at anything before. I'd never been helpful to anyone before. And here I was lugging an Ikea bag of yoga mats to a domestic violence shelter. A local kid who had started to hang with drug dealers and petty thieves started coming around the studio. I taught him to handstand and one day he led, all apropos of nothing, a meditation at the end of class. A young woman sent me a thank you card from a treatment centre. Another confided an unsafe living situation and we called a hotline together. I taught in church basements and jails and several commercial yoga studios. I wrote blogs and articles about yoga. I attended every training I could find. Teaching wasn't a dream job, it felt like a responsibility. And I had become, uncanny miracle, a responsible person. I found myself sitting at a table at a chamber of commerce meeting. I was invited to speak to high school kids and to serve on non-profit boards. 'Who am I to teach?' I once asked a mentor. He looked at me, then back down to the dishes he was washing. 'Who are you not to teach?' he asked. Later, after the Sandy Hook shooting, I asked how I could possibly teach that night. I bleated at him across a thousand miles while holding my head in my hands. 'It's okay, Karin', he said: 'No one ever said you have to teach.'

This is what I mean: I have had teachers who gave me riddles and platitudes, but they did it in a way that was personal, intimate, in response to a genuine question. The same guy gave me two different answers, but it's not that he was a hypocrite. He heard the questions inside my questions, the ones I didn't know I was asking. In the first situation, I was expressing self-doubt. In the second, I doubted yoga's ability to deal with an immediate crisis. He parsed the one issue from the other because they are different things. I did open the studio that night. We lit candles. We cried.

Certified yoga teachers who have only ever come up through teacher trainings have never had that kind of support.

My teachers washed dishes with me and answered my questions with better questions.

They left the answers up to me. Like a pile of dirty dishes.

WHAT IS A YOGA TEACHER?

When folks hear I teach yoga they assume I'm a fitness junkie or a ditz wearing a flower crown. They apologize for eating meat. They covertly check out my glutes. People seem surprised when I say I don't know anything about astrology or essential oils. Eyes tend to roll, especially if I light up a cigarette as we talk.

Occasionally people think I'm something like a spiritual adept. Not a monk, really. But not, not a monk, either. They confess to me. They ask me about human suffering. They assume I have a level of spiritual maturity I frankly have not got. Because I am a yoga teacher, no one knows exactly what it is that I do.

I do know some people who strike me as deeply wise. They have a little something – something that hallows their movements. I catch whispers of a stability so far inside them it smells of groundwater. Generally, these people don't take any kind of teaching role.

I also know some experts. I know one man who knows more about roses than I know about almost everything combined. Experts talk about physics or literature or baseball statistics in a soft, mesmeric way. They are still in love, and still marked by the fascinated unknowing which is the signal of love, with whatever it is that rocks their boat. 'Oh ho!' says the rose man, picking up speed in the botanical garden; 'What do we have here?'

There is a difference between being an expert and being a teacher, and a difference again between wisdom and teaching. If we drew Venn diagrams, some experts would be teachers and others wouldn't, some wise folks would be professional, and others would be unaffiliated. Expertise and teaching are not the same thing. Life wisdom isn't the same as trustworthy leadership.

'Yoga teacher', comparatively speaking, doesn't have a valid claim to either.

It turns out being a yoga teacher isn't about expertise or wisdom. Teaching yoga is simply a kind of relating.

Over the years, certain things have become clear. Many of the people who had the information I wanted – how to breathe, or yogic philosophy, or the neuroscience of trauma – were deeply flawed human beings. I often found myself learning from them but knowing I would never want to be in relationship to them. Various cults, cliques, and abuses of power moiled in the wings. As I went further, I realized many of the things I'd been told about yoga were demonstrably untrue.

Now I love a good metaphor, me. But I also believe in calling a stone a stone, and abuse abuse, and a sale a sale. Much of the yoga world flaunts its denial of historical reality, common sense, and ordinary lives.

I realized most yoga teachers were just like me: we didn't have a clue what we were doing, and yet we were put in positions that implied we did. Personal integrity and the praxis of the yoga industry were at odds. A pressure resulted.

Sometimes this pressure pushed us to faking it. Sometimes it pushed us to honesty about how little we knew, and spun us back into buying more training. But the longer I hung around, the more yoga training proved to be repetitive fluff.

Listen closely: the very places hawked as training schools or workshops proved to be smoke screens and propaganda. Sometimes they were initiated into a closed community. Often, they mingled yoga with sales of branded products. Yoga teacher training is not a route to personal or professional advancement, the two things it purports to be. Yoga teacher training is a Ponzi scheme.

I found no place for questions, confusion, or guidance in training. I found it outside of the yoga industry: in anatomy studies, say, or something like actual history. Teachers like me stopped going to studios. Instead, we got on Skype calls with a teacher across the globe. We got together in our living rooms. We sent long emails back and forth. Many of us quit.

I just never happened to quit.

Here is the second way in which I have been lucky: I never really fit into the yoga scene. I was always an outsider. It wasn't intentional, but I never fell into a cult, became a brand ambassador, or signed a non-compete agreement. I lingered at the fringes. Teachers would say something bizarre about chakras spinning in the wrong direction or the retention of semen. They would lay on my naked back with their naked sweaty torso to deepen my *pascimotanāsana*. But that wasn't important or interesting to me. I blinked and moved on.

It's not that I was smarter than anybody else. It was only that I was driven more by a need to stay alive than their promises.

I had the very definition of resilience: a web of diverse supports. I had family, 12 step sponsors, therapists. I studied brains and anatomy by auditing university courses and using a library card. I studied *Vedānta*, chant, and *prāṇāyāma* with teachers in India, over Skype. I sat with Buddhist communities and Benedictine monks. I signed up to study the *Gītā* at a local Hindu temple every Sunday night. And I never lost contact with grassroots communities. I was told about self-care by Black women who handed me Audre Lorde paperbacks decades before I stepped on a yoga mat. When I eventually got to yoga studios, I was willing to do whatever it took, but I was never isolated, a combination that seems in retrospect to have quite a bit of spin to it.

I've tried to explain this to people outside of yoga. They crumple their foreheads. 'I didn't know that', they say. They don't realize there is a gargantuan, pushy, prettified front to the yoga industry. Everybody assumes that front 'is' yoga. This front says yoga is a thing done in studios, bought by the class, and endorsed by both Oprah Winfrey and Deepak Chopra. It's winnowed down to fitness. Yoga fitness is further reduced to lengthening the hamstrings so you can do the splits.

Yoga is whispered to be ancient Eastern wisdom, but there is no discussion of history or the legacies of colonialism. Generally speaking, there aren't any South Asians in the room. You can bio-hack your way to mindful productivity, if not exactly immortality. We're told mindfulness will soothe anxiety, depression, and trauma. Often, it does, but there is no conversation about what caused our conditions.

Behind the façade there are an awful lot of get-rich-quick schemes. Or get-well-quick schemes. Or both together, in a bold neo-liberal swagger. The air is greasy with spiritual bypassing and cultism. A lack of accountability, cultural sensitivity, or coherent study distorts the air and pulls the ground from under you. You are left feeling lonely and ashamed. Self-soothing supplants any thinking about problems or genuine spirituality. Front facing, first accessed teachers tend to be newly minted and uninformed, unwitting. What is more, the yoga teachers you see are generally able to 'teach' because of social privilege, which creates a cyclical absence of diversity. Theo Wildcroft has written about the waning of the 'guru on a pedestal' model, but there remain a cadre of influencers who have such a glut of followers there is no genuine teaching involved. Teachers become content creators and students are now consumers. It's a vortex of obscured history, shady money, and missing people. There is a void of elderhood.

Perhaps most heart-breaking of all, you sooner or later realize that there is no 'real', no 'true' yoga. Yoga has meant and means things you don't believe in, would never do, things you see as wrong. Yoga means nothing. Your hands feel empty. It feels like anarchy, and it tastes bitterly nihilistic.

And yet yoga means so much to us, personally.

We might hit a point of heartbreak in recognizing the façade. It sometimes feels as if the façade is all that there is. But there is something behind it. It's us. It's me. Here we are.

THINKING CRITICALLY ABOUT TRAINING

I know this much: a child can teach yoga. I have had more profound conversations about embodiment with children than I've ever had in a teacher training module. I've also had exquisite conversations about death and *śavāsana* while teaching in a queer substance abuse treatment facility. Those folks had no investment in teacher training or hankering after enlightenment. We just lay on our backs together, mourning and transcendent.

If a child can teach yoga *āsana*, we need to rethink what we're really doing in teacher training programmes. Obviously, you don't need much anatomy jargon. Nor do you need a philosophy certificate. All you really need to teach yoga is a bit of experience and a willingness to share your experience with others.

I have, over the years, owned a yoga studio, run a teacher training, and run something called the Anti-200 hour programme. I tried very hard to make this programme not a training, but it didn't really work. Everybody called it a training anyway.

I'd tell people they were already qualified to teach on our first day. I'd prove it to them. I asked each of them to share their favourite yoga thing: a pose, a breath, a thought. Then I asked them to guide us through their least favourite yoga thing. 'Voila', I'd say: 'You are already qualified to teach!'

But yoga is also like playing a difficult instrument. No rational person would think they could teach other people to play the violin after a month of practice.

Striking a balance between these two very real and very simple truths is a pretty good way to approach yoga teaching.

We have to understand the history of teaching yoga. As I've already said, yoga was traditionally passed on by *ācārya*s, or elders. *Ācārya* means something like teacher, and it implies not only a demonstrated knowledge of a specific and limited thing, like a particular text, but a further study of teaching that thing to others. We should also understand that, traditionally speaking, much that we today consider 'yoga' was handed down through heritage: familial and cultural understandings that took place over generations. We should further understand that colonialism raises a lot of questions about both practice and teaching. For example: I as a white woman have had the privilege to study yoga philosophy from within a lineage, including vast amounts of oral teachings and mentorship not available in texts, a privilege systematically denied to many South Asians.

'Certified yoga teachers', in comparison, were invented in the late 1990s. Something called the Yoga Alliance was born, and with it the 200-hour model. It was a bare scratch minimum. The model was never intended to be the sum of yoga pedagogy or a replacement for yoga practice. Because in capitalism anything that can be sold will be mass produced, standard is exactly what the 200-hour model became. Teacher training has become the standard place to learn yoga, which is complicated if you realize that learning and teaching are two distinct things. Once we're in, we don't know what the alternative would be, and by that point we are financially and emotionally invested.

Certified yoga teachers are only ever taught *āsana*, even if lip service is given to ethics, philosophy, or lifestyle. It's weird. Spiritual and ethical words are used to lend credence to dubious physical stuff, but the spiritual and ethical words are never themselves explained. Meditation and mindfulness were co-opted from the Indian subcontinent as well, but went the way of psychology and medicine, privileging the brain to the exclusion of the body and a doctor's degree to a person's lived experience. Yogic spirituality is alternately primitivized and weaponized. *Karma* and *dharma* are exploited to abuse our insecurities and spiritualize oppression.

My arguments are not to suggest that modernizing yoga has ruined it. The goal here is not to 'go back' to yoga's roots. The *paramparā* model of lineage is heavy with casteism and patriarchy. The ancientness of yoga is no argument for its sanctity: slavery and foot binding are similarly old. Attempting to reconcile ancient understandings with the modern erases Indigenous wisdom while positing that modern science has a reality that it does not. Science is not truth but an attempt to find the truth. In that sense, I'd argue that yoga is already a science.

If a yoga teacher's credibility does not come from teacher training, and that was the end of the argument, it would be okay for anyone to do anything they want and call it yoga. We find ourselves in a crisis of faith. There is no accountability in this model.

FINDING OURSELVES

The resolution to this crisis is the crisis itself. It lies in our ability to think critically and stay present. Where, and how, do we find ourselves?

We find ourselves together, for one thing. We must keep each other safe, and we can't do it alone. We need to stop assuming trainings signify anything and instead create relationships.

If we value collaboration, we can break out of the echo chamber of the yoga industry. We can protect folks from abusers within it, but also the harmful groupthink of Hindutva, QAnon, and others. We can work with schools and mental health practitioners. We can work with science and medicine rather than positioning ourselves against them. Once we no longer have to have all the answers, we can put ourselves in relationship with people who are already doing the work. We can be in solidarity with rather than co-opt social justice movements.

We can recognize our limitations. Teacher training did not give us a comprehensive understanding of history. We lack a medical understanding of bodies. Teacher training is not a replacement for decades of life wisdom. Hard as all of that might be to admit, it's only in admitting it that we begin to articulate our scope of practice and can say, 'I don't know' without it feeling like an admission of failure. We can embrace diverse nodes of expertise and doors yawn open. Music! Science! Critical race theory! I mean if we really want to learn yoga things, we can. We just have to look outside of the industry to find it.

And we begin to uncover, slowly and fumblingly, our real values. This: this stays. And this other thing, no; this is wrong. If we don't know our own values, we have no way to evaluate the stupefying amounts of information we've come across. A hangnail becomes as important as a heart attack.

Both learning and healing are social. We heal in community because we tend to have been harmed in community. We learn who we are from one another. We must curate and protect relationships beyond specious 'registration' or predatory 'training'. Our teaching practice must have room for our grief, our anger, and our burnout.

Professionalizing often erodes our practice. It can also erode our moral centre as we get enmeshed in the hustle and the various power dynamics involved. It's terribly important that we talk about working conditions, politics, and conflicts. And it's important that we be able to name the things we love.

This is a shift from dogmatic methodology to learning. Learning asks you to participate in the process rather than be a consumer of information. What we know can become applied knowing. Our doubts and questions are validated. Our confusion becomes a starting point.

The end of learning isn't a certificate of your validity, but knowing that your validity is independent of measure. You can adapt your approach to different contexts as they arise. You can ask for help. You can tolerate unknowing. Our knowledge is resilient in the same way that people are resilient.

If we don't value learning, mistakes become existential crises. Our entire philosophy crumbles. Our career falls apart and our self-esteem withers.

Learning is related to compassion in ways that information will never be. Information makes you dependent and complicit; learning makes you independent and responsible.

This becomes a model of respect. I have been repeatedly disrespected in the course of my career. Respect comes as a terrible relief.

THINKING CRITICALLY ABOUT TEACHING

Developing relationships with our students is the most important aspect of teaching. Science backs this: students learn more and more comprehensively when they are valued for who they are over what they can or cannot do.

What if, instead of thinking of what we do as teaching yoga, we taught people *how to learn yoga*? It's a subtle change, but yoga has taught us that the subtle cracks open the world. What if we encouraged students to shop around, practise on their own, try yoga things outside of yoga class? What if we taught them how to find teachers, information, support? What if we flat out taught that yoga is neither *āsana* nor a yoga class? What if class became something co-created, participatory, one small piece of a much larger whole?

This doesn't happen if students have the impression we're giving yoga to them, literally or obliquely, through *śaktipat* or demonstration. We have to explain that they are not learning yoga through mimicry or proximity. Yoga teaching shouldn't be performance, indoctrination, or saviourism. The student–teacher relationship is the crux of pedagogy not because the teacher is important, but because it is the relationship that creates a context in which learning begins.

I read a cool mathematics thing the other day. This is huge for me, as a high school dropout and someone who won't do long division without a calculator. This is what I read: triangulation is determining the relationship between two things by means of a third. I wiggled and grinned. I thought of all the triads in my arsenal: bones and gods, spirals and nonbinaries. But mostly this one: student–teacher–yoga. The relationship between student and teacher is yoga. The relationship between student and yoga is a teacher. The relationship between teacher and yoga is a student. That is: if we take the teacher mantle, then yoga is defined and delimited by the student. But of course, we don't have to take that mantle, or not always. If we are also a student – because we've already established learning is vital – then our ongoing yoga is defined by having teachers. That is a Desikachar riff, excuse me and thank you.

I celebrate the fact that students outgrow me, and often leave yoga entirely. One student remembered how much she loved singing in the church choir and went back to it. I've known folks who practise hard through a rough patch in their lives, and then go back to golf. Forgive me, but I don't think I failed. I think the yoga did what it needed to do.

'The goal of yoga is not more and more and more yoga', I say all the time. 'The goal of yoga is you.'

I QUIT

I could say I'm quitting for all the reasons you will read about in later chapters of this book. I've certainly grappled with each of them. But that isn't it. As the authors will make clear, these aren't reasons for quitting so much as they are the questions that keep us going. They are vital signs.

I'm quitting for myself.

I said before that no one ever told me I should go to teacher training.

True: I was never pressured by any of the communities or teachers I knew at the time. But I was aware of the tone, the presence, of that narrative. It was in the air I breathed.

But that isn't what made me go. One night in the first summer of my sobriety, I was sitting in a lawn chair next to a bonfire. I was talking to a friend. I was trying to tell him what yoga felt like, what was happening to me. The dark helped. We didn't have to look at each other because we could both look at the fire. I mentioned wanting to go to training and then fell quiet. He flicked his cigarette into the fire, put his feet on the ground and his hands on his knees before standing up. He walked off into the wider dark. From behind me, he said, 'Well then, I think you should go.'

Going to training, being a teacher, were the right things for me to do then. Have you ever continued to do a thing because you were praised for it? Have you ever gone on doing that thing, even if it's no longer good for you?

As a little girl, I wanted to be a writer. I wanted to write when I was three, when I was 16, and when I was 40 years old. I've always had myriad, complicated, tangled, and painful things keeping me from actually doing it. A terror of falling apart. Staggering perfectionism and crooked self-esteem. I lacked means and I lacked support. But here I am; here we are.

Writing probably won't make me any money. But I figure this is a third way in which I've been lucky; since I've been a yoga teacher for a very long time, I know how to make broke work.

We can do that, I mean. Make broke things work. We've been doing it all our lives.

2 —

FALLING SHORT OF KNOWING

Donna Farhi

Donna Farhi has been practising yoga for over 46 years and teaching since 1982. She is the author of four contemporary classics: *The Breathing Book* (1996), *Yoga Mind, Body & Spirit: A Return to Wholeness* (2000), *Bringing Yoga to Life: The Everyday Practice of Enlightened Living* (2005), and *Teaching Yoga: Exploring the Teacher–Student Relationship* (2006), which is a curricular text for teacher training worldwide.

Her fifth and most recent book, co-authored with Leila Stuart, *Pathways to a Centered Body: Gentle Yoga Therapy for Core Stability, Healing Back Pain and Moving with Ease* (2017), is becoming the go-to text for yoga teachers, therapists, and somatic practitioners. The book is grounded in personal experience. In April 2017, Donna fractured her pelvis in two places as a result of a serious riding accident. Her lengthy rehabilitation has given her extraordinary insights into the profound consciousness of the body and its ability to heal.

We asked Donna if she could write for us a personal reflection on 'critical thinking for yoga teachers' because her long career is a case study in integrating new and often difficult knowledge into teaching. Like Karin Carlson's piece, what we received is a personal reflection on the journey into teaching, learning to trust inner wisdom, learning through experience, and above all, learning to question received wisdom from powerful and highly respected authorities of all kinds.

Donna also maintains a well-deserved ambivalence to teaching yoga as an industry. For Donna, there is more power in embracing 'not knowing' as a pedagogical process, as well as a personal practice. With help, she says, a yoga teacher can provide students with space and resources to encourage personal enquiry, leading when necessary, but allowing enough space for students to feel both safety and bravery. Donna's journey suggests that for at least some of us, some of the time, we are able to create a space of sanctuary, holding back both commercial imperatives and therapeutic expectations long enough for students and teachers to relate more authentically through yoga. Together, these two pieces are the perfect foundation for the sections that follow, written by two of the most accomplished writers on yoga that we know.

The most insightful moments in practice, and in teaching yoga, have come to me when I have stopped thinking and seem to be held in the potency and fullness of an invisible field that I shall call 'intelligent not-knowing'.[i] Paradoxically, it has taken decades of rigorous academic study, experiential practice, and the crucible of teaching many others to withstand the still immediacy of this place inside myself and to be able to give up all pretext of definitive answers. For it is in this luminous quietude that so much that is helpful, nourishing, and generative takes place.

While at first daunting, it can be a relief for a teacher to lay down the heavy burden of being the expert who answers another's questions with absolute authority. When we answer questions out of hand, we may be usurping the student's process of enquiry and disenabling their ability to arrive at their own ideas and possibilities. Many students have told me that hearing their teacher say, 'I don't know' or 'I'm not sure' or phrases such as 'Let me consider this and come back to you' have served to ground their perception of their teacher as human and limited. This revealing of one's humble humanness does not diminish the power of a teacher or undermine the student's confidence in the teacher's competency. On the contrary, such honesty helps to build relationships built on the mutual understanding that all living processes are complex, interwoven, and contextual and that formulaic answers provide but a mirage of simplicity. In truth, the answer to most questions is 'It depends'; on the person, the situation, the context, and the time in which an experience arises. Working with students in a dynamic process of shared enquiry that allows for co-learning now feels absolutely natural and easeful to me, but training others to teach in this way is a challenging task that takes time and patience.

---

i   This, importantly, is an unmediated process: 'without anyone or anything intervening or acting as an intermediate'. University of Sussex, 'Unmediated', n.d., www.sussex.ac.uk/languages/files/awg/glossary.html#ref21.

A huge part of that challenge is addressing automatic assumptions that have dominated the yoga tradition and now the yoga industry.

For the promise of most yoga teacher training programmes is to arrive at certainty and to confidently set forth, method under one arm, the validation of lineage under the other; and with conviction to deliver to nascent devotees a quick and efficient path to that same certainty. This desire for certainty and the apparent security that it evokes is understandable given the terrifying immensity of that great animal of life that we are all riding. We humans have a compelling need to bend every situation, no matter how precarious, towards certainty. We should not, however, confuse the *increased confidence* that is necessary for acquiring competence and capacity with the hubris of certainty. Certainty denotes the conclusion or end of a journey. It implies having reached something solid, effable, and final. Confidence, on the other hand, acts to leverage our next exploration, experiment, or adventure into the unknown. Confidence may even give us the capacity to live with our uncertainties without being overwhelmed by them. Pedagogic models that tread the well-worn path towards immutable certainty provide models for training teachers that are easy to deliver and replicate. This has huge advantages and financial implications which will be obvious to anyone who knows how to work a calculator. But such models do not give the practitioner/teacher access to a means of deepening and broadening their own understanding. Nor do such models prepare teachers to work adaptively with the messiness and complexity that is a human being.

A CIRCUITOUS PATH LEADING BACK TO SELF

My own journey towards a path of practice and of teaching that honours intuitive wisdom has been circuitous. Long before I knew that yoga could be a competitive sport or that my personal practice should be captured and commodified for a public audience, I was at the age of 16 practising daily alone in my bedroom, a well-worn copy of *Richard Hittleman's Yoga: 28-Day Exercise Plan* (1969) on the floor beside me. In the seven years that followed, I practised religiously, mostly to manage the anxiety and depression I felt in an environment that was equal parts unsafe and stultifying. When I left home at the age of 17, my practice went with me. During those seven years of unguided practice, I do not recall a single instance of feeling strain in my body or of being injured through the practice of yoga. I have no recollection of feeling any sense of striving or of 'giving my body instructions'. This practice was entirely unmediated and while crude, was perhaps some of the most authentic yoga I can claim to have experienced.

All of this changed after attending my first Iyengar yoga class. Within a few months of receiving formal instruction, I incurred one of the worst injuries of my life, rupturing a disc in my neck, an acutely painful injury that was entirely preventable and one that would have lifelong consequences. How the injury occurred was a lesson itself in the dangers of a pedagogic model in which the 'teacher knows best'. Upon feeling painful sensations in my neck, I wisely came down out of headstand, only to be directed to go right back up and to proceed into an advanced twisted variation. Like so many naïve students, I believed that the teacher's insight was greater than my own, even though my own nociception[i] was telling me to get the hell out of that pose! I proceeded, injury in tow, into a two-year training programme at the Iyengar Yoga Institute of San Francisco, convinced that this gold standard course would be my ticket to truly understanding and perfecting the practice of yoga. As I observed the popularity of the method and the ravenous appetite Americans had for workshops, I also hoped my certification would lead to some form of financial freedom. While I learned many useful things during my time at the institute, and became proficient at practising advanced postures, as time went on, I felt a growing chasm between the organic three-dimensional fluidity and interiority of my own practice and the regimented hieroglyphic rigidity with which I was supposed to teach. Any personal evolution or new insight I might be gaining through my own interoceptive awareness, academic study, or exposure to the cutting-edge somatics available in the Bay Area was now filtered through the lens of whether it tied *exactly* with the method; a method that was now remotely controlled via a guru who lived in India and relayed through an inner circle of senior teachers.

I had for some time felt a deep conflict with the cult-like dynamics of the organization and its increasing obsession with a rigid mould into which both students and teachers must bend, squeeze, or forcibly render their bodies. It was inevitable that something would have to give. That moment came unexpectedly in the summer of 1987 when I was physically assaulted by B. K. S. Iyengar at the first Iyengar Yoga Conference held at Harvard University in Boston. A full accounting of this event would take us off course but suffice to say that it would take many decades to comprehend the symbolic nature of having one of this century's most influential yoga masters stomp his heel into the soft belly of my abdomen and strike, with premeditation, my ovary.

---

i   Proprioception of pain.

It would take a long time for me to heal from this experience. But more importantly, it would take the benefit of hindsight to understand that being pinned painfully under the foot of a raging male yoga guru was ultimately not personal to me. One day you wake up and realize that the foot of thousands of years of patriarchy is literally standing on you, demanding that you submit to its dictates. That it is not one man, or one method, but the multigenerational force and collective consciousness of centuries of suppression of feminine wisdom and intuition.

One would assume that such an experience would call for immediate annexation. That it was not gives cause to consider the powerful grip that lineage can hold over one's psyche. From Boston I travelled onwards to study in England and India (globe hopping from one psychopathic yoga teacher to another in a state of disassociation) and returned to San Francisco, finances completely emptied, where I descended into a profound depression. A year later, I would reveal to my unitarian minister what had happened to me in Boston and for the first time heard my experience described as *abuse*. Up until that moment, the submission, humiliation, and physical assaults that I witnessed had become so normalized that it was not until I left the institute that I had the strength to know what I already knew. I was also completing my bachelor's degree under the academic mentorship of George Araki, the then director of the Institute for Holistic Health at San Francisco State University. He was convinced that I was onto something with my reconstruction of yoga as primarily unmediated and that it was imperative that I 'not skip onto someone else's track'. 'Follow the scent you are sniffing like a bloodhound!' When I completed my degree, summa cum laude, I considered entering a masters or doctorate programme at another institution because following that scent into the dark recesses of my own psyche and intuition was a frightening and terribly lonely experience. During an interview with the dean of a prospective school, he announced that 'there is absolutely nothing for you at this school'. He tried to console me with an analogy and story about Schoenberg the composer. 'He did his best work *before he figured it all out and began codifying it into a technique.*' I left his office and walked for hours and hours through the city streets, overwrought by the awareness that I was, simultaneously, completely lost and completely free.

Lest it be construed that one awakens to inner truth in a singular epiphany, it was my experience that finding one's footing in the vast territory of possibility is a gradual process periodically expedited through the intervention of seminal thinkers, collegial exchange, and caring mentorship. In a shared-enquiry model for teaching, it is also the willingness of our students to experiment *with us* so that we can progress from rough-hewn teaching to something more refined. In my early years of teaching, I was often stabbing in the dark as I struggled to articulate my ideas, but I had the company and compassion of loyal students who were excited by and willing to participate in these adventures. Still, when the only representations of yoga that exist and are deemed authentic operate with the brutal efficiency of a communist regime in squashing dissent, support for an alternative is often sparse, and scathing criticism abundant. To leave can feel like being cast into outer darkness. One night in the depths of a prophetic dream I found myself crawling along the floor of the ocean, too afraid to swim in the deep water and wanting to feel some solidity under my body. Midway through that ocean crossing, the water darkened to impenetrable sightlessness. I could see no way forward and only the desire to turn and go back to a known shore. Beside me, one of my spiritual mentors, who I could not see but whose presence I could feel said, 'Don't be afraid, I am with you.'

As I began to share in my teaching a practice informed through the innate and natural intelligence of the body (yet also grounded in the science of anatomy, kinesiology, and the study of human developmental movement) I encountered many students who seemed to believe that there was a Big Brother watching them who had the power to censure their every move. One woman shared that what she learned with one particularly brutal yoga teacher was 'how to hate herself' after years of unrelenting corrections. This, I would discover, was not a unique experience. Students would often linger long after class had finished to tell me, warily casting their gaze about the room as if it had been wire tapped, 'What you are teaching on some level I already knew, but I was afraid to follow it.' These experiences served to reinforce for me the incredible power that these archaic pedagogic models have to stifle and suppress intuitive wisdom. Fortunately, when people are given explicit permission and encouragement to follow the guidance of their own inner reference system there is often no going back. The desire for immutable certainty is replaced with a growing confidence in navigating the dynamics of change and evolution.

Not everyone could make this radical amendment and I counselled, on more than one occasion, students who were considering suicide rather than relinquishing their certification or identification with a particular method. When you leave a dysfunctional relationship, you cannot be entirely free until you own your part in it. Put bluntly, there is often an implicit promise made by yoga organizations that adhering to the dictates of the leader and to their method will bring you professional status and the financial wealth that comes with it. The fear of excommunication and the real threat of professional and personal exile can leave teachers emotionally and financially vulnerable. My own renunciation of my Iyengar certification left me a pariah for years, with long-time hosts closing their doors to me. Unable to find sufficient teaching work to survive, I turned to writing to archive my new understandings.

Day by day I began to realize that I could do whatever I wanted (just as the great yogic discoverers had done before me...) and that there was no ancient scroll with definitive yoga postures and magical sequences that if only replicated verbatim or held long enough or performed *perfectly* with the utmost attention to *every single* detail would deliver me to that place that I'd been striving towards. One day, as poet Mary Oliver intones, 'there is a new voice which you slowly recognize as your own'[1] and discover that just like the original yogi, who woke up in a human form with human challenges, that the only way to truly understand yoga is to land inside your own idiosyncratic human bodymind and let it reveal to you what it wants, needs, and loves.[2]

When you do finally take those shackles off you may be surprised to discover that you might, for some time, feel quite lost and disoriented and that this disorientation may compel you to seek yet some other structure or method or 'way' that can ameliorate the discomfort of being in an open space with open possibilities. Or, as I have often witnessed, you may experience a 'rubber band effect' where the awesomeness of not having your experience externally contained terrifies you to the extent that you return to the hermitage of your method and recommit with ever greater zeal to its rules and regulations. You tighten the chains even further and apply for your next certification level. But if you can stay in that open space long enough to recognize what you are leaving behind, you may also be able to intuit what you are carrying forward with you. Because all that energy and discipline and tenacity can now be harnessed for some other purpose.

What happens next is crucial. If you can increase your threshold for being in the mystery, all that compressed energy and outward striving and need to please and receive approval from others can be redirected towards finding and strengthening your own inner reference system. And if, as is true for many people, your internal landscape feels like a remote, uncharted wilderness in which there are few trail markers, this is when it can be useful to have a teacher. This is when it can also be useful *not to have a teacher*, at least in the traditional sense of what the word implies. This is when having some discernment and critical thinking capacity and a fair dose of cynicism can be useful, because that sexy newly branded contemporary yoga method may be a smokescreen for yet another yoga celeb who has found 'the way' and will be filtering this through the same fusty pedagogic lens that will land you right back where you started. This reminds me of the beautiful words of Octavio Paz's beautiful translation of a poem by Dharmakīrti:

No one behind, no one ahead.
The path the ancients cleared has closed.
and the other path, everyone's path,
Easy and wide, goes nowhere.
I am alone and find my way.

Octavio Paz[3]

ALONENESS AND INNER RESOURCES

When I finally left the Iyengar method, I discovered that even the supposed renegades who were defiantly offering a more feminine and organic approach to yoga were still hellbent on converting me to their own dogmatic rendition of yoga. One teacher encouraged us all to feel free to move away from the structure of the guided practice, yet when I moved to a corner of the room to explore an alternative, he was clearly unable to conceal his rage. I could not find a teacher who could engage with me through a collaborative pedagogic approach in which I would be free to forge new ground. Ultimately, that led to a long period of practising on my own and struggling to find some way of articulating the powerful sensations and insights of my own somatic adventures for my students.

I am not sure that it is possible for a practitioner/teacher who wants to take a deep dive and be able to facilitate that deep dive for others to circumvent the solitary nature of unmediated exploration. Yet I also feel confident, based on the feedback from hundreds of students and training teachers over many years, that a shift in pedagogic model that holds the student's self-sovereignty as key can make the teacher a potent ally, providing opportunities for growth for both parties.

PEDAGOGY, ANDRAGOGY, AND HEUTAGOGY

The word pedagogy in its strictest definition refers to adults teaching children. This is an apt description of the type of learning that has infantilized generations of yoga students and teachers. In this more traditional model, it is assumed that the learner has few resources, and the teacher attempts to download their knowledge onto and into the student, often with the intended result that the student will then copy and memorize this information. This information can then be recalled verbatim in a test or examination which may require little if any critical thinking capacity. Think 'monkey see, monkey do'. And consider that erosion of critical thinking is a key component of power inequity as well as an optimal environment for abuse.

Andragogy refers to the teaching of adults. In an andragogic model, it is assumed that adults come to the table with their own rich experience and resources. In this model teacher and student can learn from each other and be enriched by each other's experiences. If you have ever felt extreme reluctance to share an observation with a yoga teacher that might counter their instruction, and if you are certain that this sharing will result in defensiveness, you most certainly are not learning in the land of an andragogic teacher.

A more contemporary term, heutagogy (based on the Greek word 'self') is defined as the study of self-determined learning. It is a student-centred instructional strategy that emphasizes the development of autonomy, capacity, and capability. In heutagogic learning the teacher provides a context for the learning but the student is integral to deciding the path of his or her learning experience. Importantly, it is not the teacher's job to change the student or to decide the nature of that change nor the pace at which it occurs. Rather the teacher's job is to provide an optimal context where change can occur when a student feels readiness, desire, and the ability to integrate new understandings.

In a heutagogic framework of learning, the map can never replace the experience of exploring the territory. While the teacher may be able to describe where the trails are and what you might experience, it is not until you are walking the trail yourself that you come to know it. The teacher's job is to increase the student's confidence, capacity, and skill base to explore that territory. In this approach to teaching, the teacher attempts to provide a context, usually in the form of guided enquiry where you, the student, can acquire ever increasing degrees of grounded sensitivity. In something so basic as the practice of a yoga posture, breathing technique, or meditation, you may then become the expert in knowing how long, how deep, how often (if ever) you may wish to be in this form or practice. You will come to know whether it is relevant or not to your needs. Through that accumulating experience you may adapt and tailor practices to fit your individual needs, circumstances, and proclivities. And because you are a changing biological entity, those needs will change. As you change, this adaptive and responsive intelligence and approach to working *with* yourself rather than *on* yourself may serve you for many years to come whether you have a teacher at your disposal or not.

Heutagogic learning is the territory of those who are inclined towards self-guided education, also known as autodidactism. This can serve us on and off the yoga mat, because in many instances we will not be able to find someone to help us. After a traumatic riding accident that fractured my pelvis in two places, it was this firmly established ability to self-guide that allowed me to develop an intelligent rehabilitation programme. When attending the government-appointed physical therapy sessions repeatedly set back my progress, I invited a government assessor to decide if my own rehabilitation programme was a viable alternative. The assessor visited my home studio, eyes agog at the many pieces of equipment and the catalogued daily practice sessions. Based on this the government agreed to cover my loss of income during my recovery and to allow me to manage my own rehab. A vast sensory memory bank acquired over 40 years of personal practice together with a sound understanding of the body's structure gave me unique insights as to how to both avoid surgery and restore my mobility.

THE TRUISM OF TEACHER

It is a truism that a teacher is a teacher for the very reason that they *do know* more than the students they work with. It's perfectly reasonable for students to seek out teachers with the highest qualifications, experience, and competence. If I wish to go river rafting down a dangerous canyon, I want to know that the captain of the boat has the qualifications to guide that trip safely. Similarly, if I am studying how to train a young horse, I would seek out an equestrian instructor who has the depth of experience to help me do so in a way that decreases my risk of harm. In the same vein, many yoga practices are strong medicines: they have the potential to heal and inherent potentials also to harm. *Āsana* practice can be a powerful way of rebalancing and strengthening the body; but when used incorrectly it can also pull the body apart. Breathing practices and techniques such as *yoga nidrā* can provoke powerful emotional release and integration of traumatic experiences; used indiscriminately these same practices can destabilize an already fragile nervous system. For these reasons, it is important that yoga teachers have the necessary training and experience to be able to guide their students in a way that decreases potential harms. But more importantly, teachers need the necessary experience to potentiate and expedite whatever benefits yoga practice might bring.

There *are* situations in which students do not make good choices and in those situations it's important that teachers show leadership in overriding imminent harm. Such students ignore direct felt experience because they do not trust their own perception. Whatever natural insight they might once have had has been taught out of them. Their identity and sense of self may have become fused with an allegiance to a method or lineage, or to an idealized concept of the body. One of the most powerful things we can do in such a circumstance is to gradually tease out the nature of this allegiance so it can be seen for what it is. This takes time, sensitivity, and compassion. But in the immediate instance it may also require a teacher to veto the student's choices.

Unconscious allegiances can include the imperative to follow a method to the letter even when our inner perception tells us otherwise. This may include following a teacher's instructions even when those instructions are inappropriate given what we know about ourselves. Culturally, we are all influenced by the pressure to conceal our own ageing process. For teachers this can be particularly treacherous territory when their financial security relies on being able to perform physical practices and sequences that may have already caused physical degradation. The more honest and transparent a teacher can be to their own process the more likely this creates a resonant field for students to embrace themselves just as they are.

SAFE PLACE, BRAVE PLACE

Just as a teacher might need to intervene when a student may be making a poor choice, in a shared-enquiry pedagogy, the student also has the potential to challenge the teacher. The willingness to listen to our students means that there are inbuilt safety mechanisms that keep both student and teacher safe. But more than that, the safe place that is where we learn also becomes a *brave* place where we trust and can express our needs, our differences, and our discoveries with one another.

This requires that a teacher be willing to be evaluated by his or her students and, if possible, to regularly receive peer review. In this context, negative feedback becomes an essential way of identifying unsound practices, poor teaching techniques, and insensitive communication. This information gives the teacher something tangible from which to create an improved iteration of their work. At the time of writing, I have two senior students who are peer reviewing many of my classes as I am peer reviewing theirs. This is done in the spirit of friendship, with care and good humour. The underpinnings of this collaborative rather than competitive approach are the willingness to remain humble and to consider that new gains in information and scientific discovery require constant reconsideration. The acquisition of knowledge does not point to finality but rather to how much more there is to know.

FROM PERSONAL TO GLOBAL SHIFT

In many ways this may seem like a personal story. But I believe it to be a *trans*personal story that is representative of an historical and global shift towards pedagogic approaches that encourage mutual respect, shared enquiry, and the self-sovereignty and independence of students. It is also a shift towards interdependence and models of learning in which both teacher and student nourish each other and broaden each other's understanding.

What does this new pedagogy translate to in real terms in the learning space? For the teacher, it can translate to teaching with an underlying sense of ease, relaxation, and clear intention. For the student, it can translate to a liberating framework where the structure that is offered is no longer definitive, and where forms, postures, and practices become suggestions that can act as springboards for new iterations and new expressions. Together it feels like a sustainable friendship welded by a desire to know what yoga is...and can be.

HONOURING OUR SOURCES

3 ___

HISTORY – A DIALOGUE, A COMMENTARY, AND FOOTNOTES[i]

Harriet McAtee, Barbora Sojková,
Simran Uppal, and Theo Wildcroft

As we said in our Introduction, there are ample well-written guides to the history of yoga. New texts are regularly written in response to the latest research. We wanted to start this section with something more unusual and, we hope, more future-proof. While Harriet, Barbora, and Theo were teaching a course together on the 'past, present and future of yoga', a debate arose about how we approach the study of history in general, and, as is often the case for us, Simran was drawn into the ongoing conversation.

Theo began, selecting questions and writing summaries for each of the main ideas arising in the transcript of the course. Harriet and Barbora responded, and then Simran's comments enriched the text with footnotes. The result was truly collaborative and, we hope, captures the kind of conversations that often happen in real life for both teachers and historians – interwoven and circling, revealing relationships between people and ideas, between research, practice, and personal experience.

Not every such conversation will benefit from the range of skills and knowledge we were able to share. But we hope this chapter encourages every yoga teacher to think less about finding the one true source of expertise on a subject, and more about circles of trust and collaboration between specialists.

---

i   Dialogue by Harriet and Barbora. Italicized commentary by Theo. Footnotes by Simran.

Question 1: What is history? What is yoga? Why are these simple questions so complicated to answer, and why are they so important to us as yoga teachers?

The heart of this chapter lies in how we, as practitioners of yoga, connect to the ideas and experiences of heritage,[i] lineage,[ii] ancestry,[iii] and precedent.[iv] But it also speaks to all the uncertainties of status and role embedded in yoga teaching, as well as all the delicate negotiations, fraught power plays, and long and terrible histories of encounters between people and nations. 'What is history?' and 'What is yoga?' are threads that pull with them untold, silenced, and lost stories.

Harriet

My study of history and yoga have almost always run in parallel. I enjoy the liminal space of straddling two ideas, disciplines, or practices at once: how one might inform and reflect on the other, and vice versa. Even now, I often read two books at once, and my practice is split across the simultaneous exploration of somatics, *āsana* practice, and Zen Buddhist meditation. Further, as an

---

i   What do I hold that I did not make, but that makes me who I am? Is it the carrying it, or the changing it? I don't cook how my Dadiji did, but I made refried beans with a ghee tarka today.

ii   Thich Nhat Hanh sings:

And that which is transmitted
Is no less than the transmitter
And I who receive the transmission,
What am I but that which is transmitted to me.

Thich Nhat Hahn, 'Unborn and indestructible', Plum Village, 22 January 2022, https://plumvillage.org/library/songs/unborn-indestructible

I wonder what it would it mean for lineage to be not about authority, but a relationship of co-dependence. Co-creation?

iii   I wrote a poem with a stanza that goes:

Theo is good at giving care she know now I need
    silence of words richness of sounds
        she begins to sing to herself no words

sea moving as she sings I remember the seals
    in the sea did my ancestor see their ancestor
        remembering

healers sitting far from the church by water
    I ask the rocks if they are my ancestors
        they say yes of course

Sometimes I pray to my ancestors, to the sants (those who are close to truth), and to the devas, of this room and land, and far away in the rivers in Punjab.

iv   Sara Ahmed taught me to cite my sources, and so did Theo.

art historian, my particular interest was in art historiography (the history of art history), and now as a yoga teacher trainer (a teacher of teachers) I find myself again in a space of pulling back from the daily practice of a discipline to consider those 'meta' questions (which really aren't meta at all) of pedagogy, culture, and history.

What has drawn me to the study and practice of both history and yoga, I suspect, is the same set of questions, the same desire to seek understanding, connection, and place, and how that might enable me to live a more integrated and engaged life. What is history if not a way of understanding ourselves in relation to the scale of existence? What is yoga practice if not a way of understanding ourselves in relation to the scale of existence?

Most recently, when I'm asked to describe what yoga is, I offer something along the lines of: 'Yoga asks the question: what does it mean to live well?' This feels both historically accurate (yoga has always been interested in what it means to live well) and flexible (what it means to live well is subject to change, evolution, and context). There are as many ways to live well as there are yogas, indeed likely as many ways to live well as there are individuals.

Ask any yoga teacher to define yoga, and you'll likely receive a diversity of responses. For what seems like a simple question, being faced with it can suddenly feel like standing on the edge of a cliff, being asked to jump into the beautiful water below. Your stomach drops, your breath catches, and your heart feels a little tighter. Something so meaningful to you should be easy to define, surely? But the ideas feel opaque and inarticulable, your tongue feels woolly in your mouth, the words just escaping you as you try to hold them long enough to answer. These simple questions – What is history? What is yoga? – are so hard to respond to because they feel both impossibly personal and universal at the same time. It can feel as if we are being asked to speak both for the deepest, most intimate facets of ourselves, and others.

As to why these questions seem so important for yoga teachers, the cynic in me thinks it is something (everything) to do with looking to shore up our own authority and power in a society that values consumable and definitive units of information. If we can't answer these questions as yoga teachers, we can't call ourselves yoga teachers, can't sell our services, can't earn a living. Our capitalistic existential angst drives us towards an appeal to age, an appeal to authority.[i]

The practitioner in me hopes for something different. This is the 13-year-old

---

i   I hate most attempts to define 'yoga' in the same way I hate most attempts to define 'heterosexuality', because both assume that there is any 'yoga' to define. I find myself calling what I do 'movement and rest' or 'contemplation and devotion', even as my brownness garners me followers on Instagram, because I must teach real yoga. Harriet reminds me we can take words for ourselves and for our communities of practice, and stand with both feet rooted.

girl who, dislocated from the world, confused in her body, alone and seeking connection, found yoga practice for the first time. These seemingly simple questions, if we are able to hold them lightly enough, with enough curiosity and compassion, might themselves become part of our practice. Offering us avenues for deeper enquiry into our bodies, minds, relationships, world. Offering ways to understand ourselves in relation to the scale of existence. Offering ways to come home to practice, and home to ourselves.

Barbora

In the teaching of *Mahāyāna* Buddhism – the doctrinal movement that arose in India around the first century BCE and became influential in East and Central Asia – the Buddha is portrayed as employing a pedagogical device known in Sanskrit as *upāyakauśalya*, 'skill in means', or 'skilful means'. According to this view, the Buddha had a particular skill in flexibly adapting his teaching to the appropriate level of his audience, so that every single person would understand the doctrine of Buddhism, the Dharma (or *dhamma*, as it is called in Pali),[i] on their own terms. Therefore, the Buddha never gave the same teaching twice, as each of his students and hearers had individual needs on the path to Buddhahood.

The vast and complex term 'Dharma'[ii] is equally prescriptive as it is descriptive: it is not only the doctrine of Buddhism, that is, the manual on how a person should behave if they want to attain the chosen spiritual goal, but also a description of the world, an explanation of how things truly are. Telling the spiritual adept how the world works and how they should behave in it ultimately changes the world for them. Yet each hearer of the Dharma[iii] understands the meaning of the world to be something else, depending on their personal context.

Although I do not identify myself as Buddhist, my understanding of the world is profoundly shaped by these concepts. My understanding of both yoga and history comes with the realization that these terms are not static, uniform

---

i   When I hear 'dahmah', I think New Agers in Los Angeles who touch the Brahmins' feet with reverence, not just because they are Brahmins, but because they are brown, too. 'Dahmah' journalling tools for 40 dollars, casteism for the Green Party spiritual consumer.

ii   When I hear 'dharma' said as in Sanskrit I twitch because I think fascist, how 'bhakt' to most South Asians means 'Hindutva zealot who will tear down a mosque again at any moment', not the *Hanuman Chalisa* sung, big heart, British accent, round a lovely fire in Devon.

iii When I hear 'dharam', contemporary Punjabi, I hear 'stick to beat queers like 17-year-old me with', or 'stick to beat me with, tomorrow'. Punjabi Marxists have no interest in 'dharam', not just because Indian communism is so secular, but because 'order' will not free us. Barbora reminds me that yoga can mean resourcing ourselves to exist with and in complexity. Paulo Freire taught expedient/skilful means, too.

definitions but living organisms that keep changing. Not only in time and place, but from person to person. If we accept this view, the invariable and timeless narrative about yoga's history, that yoga has been around, unmodified, for millennia, ceases to make sense. It has a knock-on effect on the notion of lineage and ancestry, too. Instead of stressing the unchangeable element of lineage, it allows for individual agency and a more porous understanding of the transference of knowledge. This is not to state that the ideas of ancestry and precedent are useless when thinking about yoga. By no means. It is to accept, however, that we are not the same people as our teachers or our relatives.

What is the impact of all this on how we view yoga history? Vast, I would argue. If we, just like the Buddha, centre the individual hearer of the story, and imagine that for them, yoga is not only rhythmic movement accompanied with breath but ultimately a means to grasp the world and their place in it, we give them agency and the chance to participate in the complexity of the world. Maybe, if we centre others, we will learn to centre ourselves and our own story, history, and ancestry, too.

Question 2: What can we know about yoga, given the nature of the evidence available to us?

When we compare practices of the past to practices of the present, we find that what is now and what was then can look different, or have different intentions, or have a very different context for understanding, or be taught very differently, or any combination of the above. There is no ground state, no point of generality to reference when making such comparisons. Furthermore, practices will look different when portrayed in a single image compared to on film, or when they are represented by the only texts that have been translated, and none of these will capture the sounds and smells and the experience of being saturated by the historical context that birthed a particular āsana or prāṇāyāma. The work of the historian is one of making threads between chosen points, and such choices are never politically neutral.

Harriet

We can know that there are, and have always been, many 'yogas'. We can know (because we feel it still, don't we?) that as long as there have been humans, we have likely been asking questions of meaning, of purpose, of freedom from suffering. We can know that our many yogas have concerned themselves with these questions for as far back as we have evidence for, but this evidence is often opaque, incomplete, and marked by its absences and lacunae.

We know that the evidence we have available paints a picture of a practice dominated by high-caste men, of oppressed women and lower-caste people, of using language to exclude, and using the results of practice to reinforce power and authority. An absence of evidence doesn't mean that women or other communities weren't engaged in yogic practice, but then again (as Theo reminds me), is it an absence of evidence, or evidence of absence? This is something we cannot know.

We can also know that our many yogas have shifted and changed, evolved and transformed significantly over the course of years, cultures, geographies, invasions, colonization, and globalization. That the homogenized and white-washed neoliberal iteration of yoga within wellness culture (not to mention its close cousin, the ethnonationalist, far-right iteration) is but the latest in a long line of incarnations. We can know that the adaptability of yoga has always been there and is, indeed, one of its defining and most fortifying character-istics. We can also know that our many yogas, despite the tendency to think otherwise, have never been divorced from broader society and culture (a fact I only really fully absorbed and felt in my bones recently, in conversation with Amelia Wood).[1] And we can also know that there has always been, to borrow Sheena Sood's phrasing, a 'liberatory potential' to the practices and philosophies that yoga offers.[2]

A different way of approaching this question, perhaps, would be to ask: what can I know about yoga, given the evidence available to me? I know that my life would be significantly different, I would be different, without my yoga practice. I'm certain that my life is simpler and smoother in some ways because of my practice, and more complicated in others. I know I would relate differently to those around me, and to myself. My world would likely feel more constricted, less spacious. My body, my mind, my spirit would likely feel more con-stricted, less spacious. My yoga practice offers a set of tools I use daily, hourly, in a variety of ways to support how I travel through the world. I think it likely that practitioners of our many yogas have been using their own tools in a similar way for a very long time, both within and beyond what the evidence tells us.

Barbora

I frequently fluctuate between two extremes in my study of yoga. On one hand, I am convinced that we do not have enough evidence to completely understand what yoga was in the past; on the other hand, I believe that there is enough surviving evidence – but we don't know where to look for it and how to interpret it. The truth is probably somewhere in between.

A lot of evidence of the evolution of yoga, literary as well as visual, has been undoubtedly lost. Our understanding of the history of yoga will never be complete, especially considering the fact that much of what survives are works of only certain parts of society. Voices of many pre-modern people – women, lower social groups, followers of non-mainstream religious traditions, just to name a few – vanished and with them, their unique understanding of yoga. As researchers and practitioners, we simply have to accept that our knowledge will never be absolute.

What if I told you, however, that there is a lot of evidence that researchers simply overlook? As researchers – but also as yoga practitioners, and as human beings – we often search for what we already know, or more precisely, what we think we know. We have a pre-shaped understanding of what yoga is and how it looks, and we disregard what does not quite fit.

Why is it, for example, that most of our understanding of pre-modern yoga traditions rests on normative Sanskrit texts, written by men from privileged classes of the South Asian societies? Many times, it is because the researchers and their predecessors thought Sanskrit to be the language of knowledge, and considered texts in it to be of a special importance to the traditions of the Indian subcontinent. Nineteenth-century researchers were themselves men from privileged classes, and they looked for literature that would mirror their understanding of the world.

There are countless texts on the theory and practice of yoga written in vernacular languages of the Indian subcontinent, many equally important as the ones in Sanskrit. One could argue that there are many more people who know Sanskrit than, let's say, Avadhi or Middle Bengali, and that's why they work on it. But why is that? Why do we teach our students (in universities and yoga studios alike) that Sanskrit is the pinnacle of all yogic knowledge? Why do we privilege one tradition over the other? Why do we think that the history of one part of the world, or of one particular group, is more important than the other one?

We know that there is so much knowledge about yoga (and South Asia in general) stored in countless manuscripts, in countless scripts, untouched for centuries, yet we keep mulling over the *Yoga Sūtra of Patañjali*.[i] How come we

---

i   I'm exhausted by Patañjali in the same way I was exhausted when a white yoga teacher – who had just run an expensive and well-attended workshop on the *Hanuman Chalisa* – answered my question, saying that 'of course' she chanted it in Sanskrit. A text written in vernacular, a text written as part of a thousand voices turning against Sanskrit or simply no longer placing it at the centre. All the poems of my ancestors are in Braj Bhasha, Persian, the mediaeval dialects of Hindi-Urdu and Punjabi, sometimes in chatty folk-song, sometimes Sanskritized, how I can talk to the other they/them girlies at the Queen Adelaide, or bristle and let an Oxford degree inflect my language when a white woman pushes in front of me, outside the studio I am about to teach at. We learn languages like making swords and shields for ourselves, but they want us to forget a ploughshare is already a kirpan, and that a hammer and a scythe or a sickle house and feed us, yes, but are just as good in the fight.

trick ourselves into thinking that we know anything about yoga when we ignore large swathes of evidence? Is it because vernacular yoga traditions are not as 'pristine' as Sanskrit ones?[i] I don't know; but I do know that there is plenty of work still to be done, if we want to understand what pre-modern yoga was.

> **Question 3: In what ways does the history of yoga change, depending on what, who, and when we are asking about it?**
>
> *And here we reach the heart of the matter, remembering that the answers we find depend not just on the evidence we select, nor only the questions we ask, but also who is doing the asking, and when. Whose voices dominate the telling, and who is listening?*

Harriet

The history of yoga changes, just as all history changes, depending on the context from which you are examining it. History is mutable, just as yoga is mutable. Just as two people are able to have two entirely divergent experiences of exactly the same *āsana*, two people are able to look at exactly the same evidence and come to two very different conclusions. This is the nature of subjective experience, and trying to suggest otherwise is to try and deny our very humanness.

In fact, this is easily one of my main issues with much of yoga (both pre-modern and modern); it is often consumed with getting away from our humanness. Subsuming, sublimating, transcending it until we are pure, until we can do superhuman feats with our limbs, until we stop menstruating, until we don't need our bodies, until we don't need other people. Quite frankly it brings tears to my eyes and makes my skin crawl.

One of the most relieving things I have ever heard someone (Judith Hanson-Lasater) say to me was this: 'How very human of you.' So I suppose I'm interested in asking the human questions about the history of yoga: what did yoga look like in communities? In relationships? What does yoga do for people whose voices are less heard? For those who are less seen? How does it feel to know what I can about yoga, and to carry both the heartbreak and the joy of that knowledge into my practice and teaching? How does yoga itself change when these are the questions we ask of it?

---

i   There are so many texts I want to read but can't because it would take me a day to decode a page, and again some white man has commented on Patañjali.

Barbora

The deeper we look in history, the less human and more mythical its protagonists become, and their teaching mystical and seemingly profound. History, and by extension yoga, becomes almost a blank canvas onto which we can project our ideas based on our positionality. In a way, it is yet another nod to the Buddha's concept of 'skill in means': each of us understands the world on their own terms.

There is a paradox, however. Although each of us carries a unique understanding of yoga's history, some of these understandings have a bigger magnitude than others. Some stories about yoga and its history – those told by the Western scholars versed in Sanskrit or high-class Hindus, for example – have a lot of friction. They stick onto and cover and erase stories of marginalized groups, such as Dalits, Sikhs, Jainas, women, disabled communities, the LGBTQA+ people, and all of those South Asian communities who live away from their ancestral lands and face violence daily. I want to fill this page with their names and their unique understanding of what yoga is, but I also wonder, would it be enough?

In a previous version of this paragraph, I naïvely wrote that to honour the idea of humanness we have to make sure that we honour both the stories that are told repeatedly as well as those that are 'missing' from the usual discourse.[i] Now, months after first writing the paragraph, I am reading it again, together with Simran's comments and footnotes. The second part of the sentence seems utterly nonsensical now, and it is Simran whose comments shake up my myopic understanding, gently but firmly. What was I thinking when I was writing that? How could we even honour stories that are not there, that are being erased? Who is doing the honouring, and who is doing the erasing? Is 'honouring' enough, and what does it even entail? We should do much more than that: we should change the paradigm in such a way that no one is worried about sharing their stories in the first place, and educate those who listen to them.

---

i   I dream of a world where people of colour can be more ambitious. Not in a Beyonce 'we teach girls to shrink themselves' way, although also that, but because 'Representation matters!' feels like the death of a hope every time. Our histories and the stories we see ourselves living are crucial, because they help us feel human, but what do we think our grandparents were doing when they sat safely around each others' living rooms, talking and eating? It is not just the desire to occupy the violent mainstream, but the lack of dreaming of a world where the politics of representation would be a droplet in a river, where the river is huge liberation and freedom. Redistribute Murdoch's property. Nationalize The Walt Disney Company, net worth c. 150 billion dollars. End the colonial occupation of Puerto Rico, and we might find that the need for think pieces about the new *West Side Story* movie has diminished. Money and imperial power are what control our stories; burn the violence at the root, or tell stories that inspire us to do so.

Question 4: In what ways and which contexts has yoga been a force for change and revolution?

The history of yoga is contested precisely because of the usages to which people put yoga in the present.[i] *History matters, not just to honour what was, but to honour who we are, and who we can be.*

Harriet

Yoga has always been used as a force of change and revolution – look at how it is being used now. It has never been divorced from the political, the social, the transformative. This has sometimes been for good, and sometimes for harm. Yoga accumulates power, and as Jivana Heyman says, 'Spiritual power, without service, is just power.'[3] Here we come to reckon with the realization that without a framework of service, without context, without perspective, the 'power' we attain through yoga practice can be put largely to any means we desire. It can be used to reinforce privilege and shore up oppression, or it can be used to fuel communities of care and liberation.[ii]

Barbora

If yoga is ultimately a means to living well, as Harriet said in one of her previous answers, it entails that it is a force for change. Since its earliest history, yoga has been an art of transformation:[iii] of one's own self, body, immediate community, the world. The microcosmos as well as the macrocosmos.

Living well is a learned skill, especially in our late-capitalist society. We are often told to prioritize our individual wellbeing, to consume, to own. Our attention has become a commodity, as Julia Bell says aptly in

---

i   There are four plants on my desk; two in great big plastic pots, one in a glass jar, and one in a little ceramic pot, with loose soil around a spiral of roots, that takes its water from the air. The desk is dark brown leather and wood, with little gold leaves impressed in rows around each section. I am sitting on my bed and writing and looking at my desk, with the window to the rest of London behind me, and I am reminded how I have found ways to fight, and how storytelling is one of them.

ii   I am editing a monthly newsletter to the members of the Yoga Teachers Union. 'Communities of care and resistance' is a phrase that comes into my everyday, from Sivanandan, from disability justice writers, and from feminist organizers. Really Theo is the person who first explained the concept to me, and I see it forming through the webs Harriet weaves through Oxford, silvery and strong, spider silk passing through walls till it meets me here in Hackney, spider silk caught in the light except it has its own glow.

iii   I have realized I do not want to transform anything in myself. I want the world to transform, so I can exist as I am, and be safe, and for the same to be true of everyone I love, and everyone I do not love. I resent the work of adaptation, even as I feel it becoming easier to live every day. There is no work we need to do on ourselves, other than to meet the landscape of our bodies – whatever parts feel like home. The rest is healthcare policy.

her book *Radical Attention* (2020).[4] Yoga, in both its contemporary and pre-modern form, challenges this. It offers a change of pace, or it can, if one looks for it. A change of perspective. One does not necessarily need to leave society and live in a cave until you dissolve your mind in the state of *samādhi*; a mere step outside of one's own habits and comfortable routine is often enough to start a small change. From my personal experience, a personal change usually translates into how we act towards the world (I am too much of a child of 90s post punk/riot grrrl movements; *osobní je politické*, that is, 'the personal is political', was a slogan I wrote on my tote bag with a Sharpie when I was 16 and it has stayed engraved in my mind until today).[i]

Question 5: How can yoga teachers best represent the vast history of yoga when teaching?

Partly, I hate that we are asking the question. It speaks to an impossible task: the condensing of an ocean of context into a soundbite or a lesson plan. But who else is better placed to tell the story of yoga to its students, at least in the first instance? Our duty, then, is to tell that first story in a way that signposts students to more, and does not steer them into dogma or fantasy. When we give a linear timeline for yoga, there's always the possibility of students thinking that reality was as neat. When we talk about yoga's history as a river or a tree, we give an impression of something inexorable, natural, with universal roots. When we talk about it as a weave, we emphasize harmony over conflict, and so on. Our ideas of the past can be complex and right, versus simple and wrong (or any mixture of these!).[ii]

Harriet

I think the beginning of this journey is for yoga teachers to (re)educate and (re/un)learn what they think they know about history in general, and the history of yoga in particular. Confusion, anger, existential anxiety, imposter syndrome, and doubt are all very common and entirely reasonable responses to having the historical rug pulled out from underneath you. This is keenly

---

i   I wonder how I make myself vulnerable by writing, but remember how we stir our prasad with a sword.

ii   I think of a piece of yarn, a single line. A crochet hook and a few hours turns it to weave, still a single line, the way a loom brings separate threads together. Frayed threads look like root fibres. A river looks like a tree lying on its side, tributaries, branches, bowls of flowers offered at sunrise like blossoms. Could the Thames look like a London plane tree, or the Ganges like a bodhi tree? How is a river like a piece of yarn – halfway spun, pulling water from the soil, how the spin pulls the fibres into itself?

felt by yoga teachers in particular, because many still draw much solace and authority from the historicity of the practice. My advice is to seek community and connection with peers and trusted teachers. These feelings, questions, and re-learnings are best worked through by discussion, communication, and the sharing of experience.

And don't be afraid about revisiting and returning to the same questions or the same material. Even now, no matter how much I feel like I've let go of my internalized ideas about the authenticity, historicity, or hierarchy of yoga, I still find new corners and spaces of my mind to shine a light on. I do this by talking with peers, listening to their ideas and insights, by sitting in on lectures even when I feel like I'll know all the content, by reading (and re-reading) articles and books, by listening to podcasts. The project of learning, re-learning, un-learning is never complete, and never linear.

You will reach a moment where your heart swells and the need to share your learning with others feels urgent and necessary. When you feel that swell, that whisper to share, that excitement, then you can be mostly certain that your sharing is coming from a genuine space. So do share, with an attitude of awe, humility, and curiosity. Be mindful of accurately reflecting your positionality, citing your sources, and sharing your process. You'll often hear me uttering phrases like 'I was reading the other day...' or 'recently I've been really interested in the idea of...' So share what you've learnt not only in the context of the broader history of yoga, but also in the context of your learning history. Share your reading lists, podcast recommendations, quotation sources. Be generous with your learning. The other side to this is: be honest with your students (and yourself) that new pieces of information come to light. Try to not erase these past iterations of yourself, but hold them close and set them down tenderly.

Allow the mutability and multiplicity of yoga(s) to be a source of excitement and joy for you and your students. Allow it to be something that broadens your definition and understanding of what it means to practise, of what practice can look like, feel like, and achieve. Share that yoga has meant many different things over many different times and cultures, and that the yoga we practise today is a synthesis, a patchwork, a tapestry, a weaving of many different traditions, ideas, modalities, and methodologies. Share that we should be wary of claims to 'truth' or 'authenticity' or 'ancientness' – that these terms all too often indicate an agenda, a prescription, a constriction. Encourage your students (and yourself) to think critically and carefully about the sources of information, the position of its purveyors, the history of its reception and utilization. History has a history too.

But mostly I think, take solace in the fact that there is a vast, interconnected web of people trying to do their best to offer us new, expansive, and representative histories of yoga. These histories may not always be comfortable for us to encounter at first, but perhaps the time has come for us to be okay with being a little uncertain, a little uncomfortable. Reflect on your own relationship with not-knowing. Allow yourself to find freedom in saying, 'I don't know,' and use that as a foundation not to shirk the responsibility of education, but to move forward with curiosity and openness to what you may find.[i]

Barbora

This question massively depends on the context. Coming back to the Buddha, each of us has unique needs when learning about a certain topic. There is no 'one size fits all'. If you worry about misrepresenting the history of yoga, it might be helpful to think about whom you are going to be addressing. Are they a fellow yoga teacher or a student who has just taken their first ever class? I am sure your explanations would differ, as would the figures of speech you would use, or the metaphors Theo is alluding to.

More crucially, however, what are you teaching? I would argue that if it is a general yoga class, there is not so much to worry about. The majority of your students do not come to your class to learn about the vast and complex history of yoga; they come to move and experience their bodies. Teaching a specialized workshop on the history of yoga is a completely different beast. Perhaps, however, the common principle that connects both general classes and specialized workshops is authenticity and honesty. Being honest that this is your version of the history of yoga might make your students curious about what their own version looks like.

---

i   There is so much comfort in uncertainty, sometimes. Why else would people pray, or sing the *Chalisa*? Not to transfer a Hanuman-certainty into this life, but to taste the certainty in the Rāma–Sīta story, the sureness of devotion, and come back to this life, how you are so relieved to let the front door shut behind you when you get back from a trip.

4 —

TOOLS FOR TEACHING NON-DOGMATIC YOGA HISTORY

Barbora Sojková

Barbora Sojková has a PhD in Sanskrit from the University of Oxford. Her doctorate focused on animals in Vedic literature, and her research interests include environmental humanities, the Anthropocene, and the interaction between philology and theoretical disciplines such as anthropology and animal studies. She has worked in university libraries in both Oxford and Prague and curated museum exhibitions, and is also a certified yoga teacher and guest teacher for yoga teacher training courses.

As an up-and-coming scholar who is also a practitioner and yoga teacher herself, she is well placed to bridge the gap between the often-arcane knowledge of academic historians and the yoga teaching and practising community.

For this piece, we asked Barbora to do more than discuss the history of yoga. We asked her to outline her favourite strategies for teaching that history to students in ways that are practical, sensitive, inclusive, and genuine. Above all, Barbora stresses the personal, positional, and relational contexts for sharing the history of yoga, which often get cast aside in the pursuit of absolute facts and simple answers which rarely exist. We are reminded of the maxim that knowledge about research can be simple and wrong, or complicated and true.

The difficult task of the yoga teacher is to answer apparently simple questions about the history of yoga in ways that retain a sense of the complex and evolving reality of historical research and are still accessible. To help, in this chapter Barbora sets out simple teaching and citation practices, shares her key takeaways for the history of yoga, and adds a wonderful primer of resources to guide further reading.

The 2010s saw many advances in our understanding of yoga history, driven especially by the publications of Mark Singleton's influential book *Yoga Body: The Origins of Posture Practice* (2010), numerous translations of mediaeval Sanskrit yoga texts by James Mallinson, as well as a joint effort of these two authors, the now indispensable textbook of premodern yoga texts called *Roots of Yoga* (2017).[1] Academically rigorous yet accessibly written, these and many other works by equally talented scholars have sparked many conversations about the evolution of contemporary yoga practice amongst researchers as well as practitioners, and opened a new chapter in teaching, studying, and researching yoga history.

Since their publication, the landscape of teaching yoga history has changed tremendously. Numerous yoga teacher trainings now dedicate much more time to history and philosophy teaching than ever before, often using the above-mentioned books in their curricula. In addition, we can observe a change in the style of teaching: in many cases, scholars, scholar-practitioners, and academically oriented facilitators (just like myself) have taken the place of inspired gurus in teacher trainings and other courses, bringing different values and teaching methods.

Many accredited teacher trainings follow the standards of international yoga associations such as Yoga Alliance or the British Wheel of Yoga when creating their curricula. Whilst these associations prescribe rough guidelines, such as the key areas of study or the time allowance for each, there is a lack of discussion about how to teach yoga history and philosophy in the first place. The standards, as well as content itself, vary from training to training: some trainings will include, for example, only a basic session on the concepts of *yama* and *niyama*, whereas others run detailed classes on everything from the Vedas to colonialism or cultural appropriation, using various forms of teaching practices.

This chapter aims to offer practical tools for teaching yoga history in the context of a yoga teacher training. Whilst it talks predominantly about history, it is also applicable to the whole field described by Yoga Alliance as the 'Yoga Humanities', that is, history, philosophy, and ethics. It is, suffice to say, neither a summary of yoga history nor a bibliography of teaching sources. Equally, it is not a guide for how to integrate one's understanding of yoga history and philosophy as a general yoga teacher, or how to represent this information to students in general movement classes. My aim is to introduce how to teach yoga in a non-dogmatic way, prioritizing evidence, inclusion, and accessibility. I will start this chapter by explaining some strategies I have been using myself, followed by suggestions on teaching or discussion topics.

STATE YOUR POSITIONALITY

If there is a single thing I would like my readers to take away from this piece of writing, it is this: the way we narrate history shapes the present and future, and it is, in turn, greatly influenced by our position in society.

This concept is called *positionality*: a notion that 'acknowledges that we are all raced, classed, and gendered, and that these identities are relational, complex, and fluid positions rather than essential qualities'.[2] Openly acknowledging our positionality is perhaps the most important guideline when teaching any form of yoga: letting people know who we are and what are the goals of our teaching and learning will help everyone to understand the reasoning behind your teaching.

I am a white, Central European woman from a working-class background. I grew up in Prague, in the post-communist Czech Republic, and as a first-generation student, I have gone on to study a doctorate in Sanskrit at the University of Oxford. I am in my thirties, a relatively long-time yoga practitioner, and a scholar of Vedic India. If you saw me in person instead of reading my writing, you would notice my gentle Slavic accent, my gender, race, age, or the shape of my body, some of which could give you a hint of why I explain certain historical facts in a specific way; other ones would, however, need more explanation. For instance, in my teaching, I tend to stress that premodern yoga is not an unchanging, static phenomenon, but a system of practices that have been shared, adapted, and reinterpreted by many religious groups of South Asia, from Hinduism to Buddhism, Jainism, and Sikhism. I emphasize this because I grew up in a certain context: although predominantly Slavic, the Czech Republic had a large German-speaking presence, Catholic and Jewish alike, since mediaeval times, and has seen a great deal of cultural adaptation and reinterpretation over the centuries. I have also lived in multiple countries and have personally experienced how one, if embedded in different contexts and speaking different languages, can adapt and reinterpret many cultural practices.

Furthermore, I am keen to stress that for the majority of history, yoga was practised at the fringes of mainstream society. I spotlight this in my teaching because my own life has been largely shaped by the influence of a counterculture. These aspects I emphasize are real and historical, but, given a different positionality, I might choose to emphasize other aspects of that rich and complex history of yoga. Other teachers could equally emphasize other aspects, shaping the broad historical narrative on the basis of their lived personal experience.

Reflecting on your own positionality in a similar way will help your teaching come from a place of authenticity, a quality that students recognize and greatly value.

CO-TEACH WITH OTHER PEOPLE

By stating your positionality, you will communicate one of the key principles of pedagogy for history: the past is shaped by the person who narrates it. Every reader always participates in a text, and co-creates it. The meaning of a text is never transferred directly from an author to a reader but is subject to unique interpretation. A text that is not being read essentially holds no meaning. Everyone has a subjective view, an agenda with which they approach a topic. This has a profound effect on the ways in which different people emphasize different aspects of history.

The best practical approach for conveying the importance of this concept and its influence on historical narratives is to co-teach classes and workshops with other colleagues. Not only will your students benefit from the multiplicity of voices in the room but it will also enable you to learn from your peers and hone your arguments. In discussion, the abstract concepts of yoga philosophy often come truly alive. Moreover, you will be able to get to know your colleagues much better, to hang out, and to access 'all these moments of down-time and serendipity and unexpected connections that lead to a different kind of conversation', as Theo Wildcroft succinctly described it in her blogpost.[3]

In my experience, the presence of multiple voices can only enhance the learning experience. For a number of years, I have been teaching yoga history and philosophy in a particular Czech yoga teacher training. This unique, two-year-long training is led by three senior trainers. All three of them have different backgrounds and specializations. As it happens, they respectfully disagree with each other (and with me) every now and then. Talking to the students in between sessions, I have realized that they value the fact that their trainers have different opinions and are able to discuss them openly, showing in practice that yoga is not a uniform, standardized practice which has to be interpreted in a singular way.

DISCUSS

Yoga history and philosophy teaching usually happens in the format of a lecture or a talk. This is, to a certain extent, inevitable: some students will have limited or perhaps no knowledge of the subject, and as a trainer in Yoga Humanities, you will have to provide some background information. If we accept the concept of positionality as the primary guideline of our teaching, however, we should beware of extensive lecturing and allow time and space for a discussion.

As teachers, we are in a position of power by default. Our voice is always the loudest one, the one to which everyone listens. By leaving time for discussions, we can hold space for everyone's voice to be heard. When teaching general classes on yoga history, I tend to start by asking people about what they already know. On one hand, this gives you a good idea of how much detail to provide in your teaching; on the other hand, by giving your students a voice from the very start, they are more likely to express themselves, ask questions, and communicate their opinions. Make sure that you always leave sufficient time for a discussion at the end of your sessions. If teaching online, breakout rooms are an excellent tool to encourage students to discuss various topics with their peers without having to speak in front of many people. In person, you can plan discussions in pairs or small groups. Do not forget that a lot of important conversations happen during tea breaks. Remember also that your students might need time to reflect and digest the material. A rest or a debrief at the end of your session can provide the same integration as a śavāsana at the end of a movement class.

NOT EVERYTHING GOES

Accepting that history is not static and shifts with various contexts is liberating. It means that where we can access historical sources, we can participate in their narratives. This approach can uplift many groups whose voices might have not been previously heard in traditional scholarship, such as women and non-binary people, the LGBTQIA+ communities, people of colour, or neurodivergent and disabled communities.[4] Equally, historical sources can be cherry-picked to support the agenda of certain groups and institutions, serving as a tool to further strengthen phenomena such as cult dynamics or totalitarian political values.

Nevertheless, historical narratives are subjective and malleable only to a particular degree. There are many historical sources – manuscripts of texts, material evidence, works of art, or orally transmitted knowledge, amongst others – that stand as witnesses to yoga history, and we have to take them seriously, trust them, and quote them truthfully. We can decide how to convey their stories and emphasize features that help us communicate our key points. We have to be mindful, however, that we do not wilfully reinterpret them for our own means. It is a hard balance to strike. I tend to use a set of reliable sources and authors, and I would recommend identifying a similar set for yourself, perhaps inspired by this book and its authors.

Another favourite approach is to show students multiple translations of a premodern yoga text side by side.[5] I let students compare the translations and experience the fact that although every translator has a very different language, goal, or agenda in mind, there are certain points – we could say a kernel of the text – that stay the same across the translations. This is a beneficial exercise, especially for those students who do not work with historical or philosophical texts on an everyday basis.

ACCESSIBLE TEACHING MATERIALS AND LANGUAGE

As a trainer in Yoga Humanities, and history in particular, your job most likely involves digesting complicated and nuanced original research, reading primary sources in translation or in original languages, and familiarizing yourself with terminology in Sanskrit and other South Asian languages. It is a long, arduous process, and it is only natural that you might be tempted to utilize as much of your work and knowledge in your session as possible. Moreover, teachers (and yoga teachers in particular) are conventionally seen as people who use complicated language full of cryptic, mystical-sounding Sanskrit terms without any explanation, and it is sometimes alluring to communicate this way.

Not only should we aim to speak in direct, not overly academic language; we should also beware of using specialized terminology without translation and/or explanation. If you want to introduce a Sanskrit or other foreign term, take the time to define it and repeatedly check with your students that they know what you mean by it. When talking about a term that is used colloquially in the yoga world, such as *karma* or *yoga*, leave space for a discussion during which students can explain their personal understandings of the term in conversation with others.

Be mindful that your students might have various learning styles and needs. Some might not be native speakers of the language in which you teach, and some might prefer to learn in an embodied way. I personally value presentations that include both text and visual sources. Be mindful that presentations can create an illusion of linearity, simplify complex material, and centre the teacher/speaker. If using them, make sure that you ask plenty of questions and leave time for discussion. I also create handouts so students can sit back and listen rather than make copious notes, and I tend to include embodied explorations (postures, meditation, rest, all taught with invitational language in mind) for those who are more geared towards embodied learning.

EMPLOY HONEST AND RIGOROUS CITATION PRACTICE

Yoga is a personal practice, and each student who comes to your classes already has a unique understanding of it and its roots. It is possible that your interpretation of yoga history, philosophy, and ethics might challenge the opinions of your students. Whilst some might agree with you, others might need time to reflect; some, however, might be left confused or truly upset by your teachings.

To alleviate the pressure and make yoga history more accessible, use a rigorous and transparent citation practice. Tell people where your information comes from. As I have already argued above, we co-create anything we read and, therefore, allowing people to access the sources gives them agency to understand the arguments on their own terms.

Reading research articles and academic monographs is a challenging, learned skill; not everyone is ready to read, for example, detailed accounts of complicated Sanskrit etymologies. If your students are keen to read the research themselves, however, share the bibliographical information with them – and if you can, the books and articles too.

It is worth pointing people primarily towards accessible sources. This means sources that are both easy to understand and easy to obtain. Again, this requires a lot of thought, as some sources might be available but not trustworthy; others factually brilliant but incomprehensible; and yet others cost more than a monthly membership in a yoga studio.

Recommend books and articles that are not misleading and that you regard as reliable sources, but can be read by non-specialists. Remember if you, like myself, teach in a different language than English but your sources are primarily in English, many of your students will not understand them. Indicating reliable sources in their mother tongue or other languages they speak will be crucial to your teaching. You might even consider translating small parts or quotes from your sources so students can access them.

Equally, many sources are not available to wide readership due to their price. Research articles often exist only behind paywalls. Academic books and edited volumes are published by specialized publishers as expensive hardbacks and are held in hardly accessible research libraries. Some scholars, more mindful of the implication of their research to the wider yoga community, now share their writings online. Nevertheless, the majority of scholarship is still inaccessible to the lay practitioner. If you have the means to access important material that others cannot, consider sharing it if you can, or think about making excerpts.

Increasingly, there are many widely available sources, such as podcasts, blogposts, or videos. These are often more accessible than printed books and research papers, and can be incredibly beneficial for people who prefer other forms of learning beyond reading. If citing them, identify which particular sources you consider reliable before you share them with your students.

To conclude this chapter, I would like to step aside from teaching practices and focus on a few elements of yoga history that I deem essential to my understanding. You might consider them to be a framework for your own teaching or topics which can be discussed with your students; I include reading suggestions in case you would like to include them in your teaching. Neither this list nor the suggested sources are by any means exhaustive. The suggestions are centred largely around premodern yoga, influenced by my academic specialization. At the end of each suggestion, I offer a list of recommended sources in the endnotes.

THERE IS NO SUCH THING AS ONE YOGA, ONLY MANY YOGAS

We know that although the Sanskrit word *yoga* (and its counterparts in other South Asian languages) has been used for a long time, it has not always had the same meaning, and the practices attached to it have differed in every single epoch. Yoga is historically a multifarious, diverse theory and practice, in a way a 'floating signifier' that gets reframed and reconstituted in various contexts.[6] It has been around at least since the later Vedic *Upaniṣads*, roughly the middle of the first millennium BCE, and more likely even longer. In the course of history, it has been a philosophical, intellectual tradition; a lived, contemplative practice; a method for reaching a certain goal; and a physical exercise. Importantly, the complicated postural forms that dominate contemporary yoga were, by and large, only part of premodern yogas. In a nutshell, yoga is a multifaceted practice which changes, just like every other living practice. Our knowledge of it is not complete, nor will it ever be.[7]

YOGA HISTORY IS MUCH LARGER THAN THE *YOGA SŪTRA*

Without a doubt, the *Pātañjalayogaśāstra*, colloquially known as the *Yoga Sūtra*, is a unique source of our knowledge of yoga, and perhaps the best-known expression of premodern yoga in general. The text is now considered to be a thoughtful synthesis of numerous strains of ancient Indian thought, especially the *Sāmkhya* philosophy, Buddhism, Jainism, and ascetic practices. In comparison with other ancient Indian philosophical texts, however, the *Yoga Sūtra* never acquired much attention from contemporary Indian philosophers, as we can judge from the few extant commentaries. Furthermore, the historical evidence of practitioners following the techniques described by Patañjali are equally scarce.

In about the twelfth century, it was identified as a key text of yoga in the *Sarvāsiddhāntasaṃgraha*, a doxographic[i] work falsely ascribed to the philosopher Śaṅkara, which amongst other topics categorized the premodern Indian philosophical schools, known as *darśana*s. Its status as a root text of the *yoga darśana* ensured its popularity with early European scholars of India who translated the text into various European languages. Inspired by the early English translations, the late-nineteenth-century religious thinker and yoga reformer Swami Vivekananda published his commentary of the *Yoga Sūtra*, called *The Raja Yoga*. This book, framing the *Yoga Sūtra* in the pseudo-scientific language of Western spiritualism, was a bestseller of its time, and came to be seen as a root text of all yoga from that point on.

This complicated history is a good reminder that the *Yoga Sūtra*, although an important expression of premodern yoga, is not the *only* one, and the influence it has in the contemporary yoga community is disproportional. Although I teach about it, I tend to emphasize that it is only one of many sources we have for understanding premodern yoga.[8]

YOGA HAS ALWAYS BEEN A SYSTEM THAT HAS BEEN SHARED ACROSS RELIGIOUS AND SOCIETAL BOUNDARIES

Although for centuries, yoga has been identified primarily with Hindu religious schools and lineages, both Brahmanical and sectarian (Śaivism, Vaiṣṇavism, and Śāktism), recent findings of yoga studies show that yoga has been a broad system shared across religious and societal boundaries. Many forms of yoga were born from interreligious dialogue: for example, in the case

---

i   Doxography is a term used usually in philosophy. It describes a text or a passage that collects and explains opinions (from the Greek word *doxa*) of other people.

of the *Pātañjala* system, mentioned above, from dialogue between *Sāṃkhya* philosophy and practices of renunciate ascetics; and in the case of mediaeval traditions of *haṭhayoga*, from adaptations and reinterpretations of Tantric Buddhism. Many religious groups created their own forms of yoga, from Buddhists and Jainas to Sikhs and *bhakti* devotees. Other religious groups, such as the North Indian Muslim *Sūfīs*, were inspired by yoga practices and incorporated them into their own teachings, as is attested in both textual and visual sources. Yoga was also not associated with a certain social class or a caste but was used across them, including groups that rejected the caste system completely.

In my experience, the permeability of yoga can be a powerful topic to talk about, both in the form of a lecture and in discussion. A good textual example is, for instance, the Arabic translation of the *Yoga Sūtra*. If possible, I would also recommend showing some examples of the striking visual evidence that demonstrates the blurry boundaries of religious denominations, such as the *Bahr al-hayat*, a sixteenth-century illustrated yoga text in Persian.[9]

EVERY FORM OF YOGA MUST HAVE BEEN, TO A CERTAIN EXTENT, A COMMUNITY-BASED PRACTICE

The written teachings usually speak about the ideal (and idealized) life of a male, ascetic yogi. It is clear, however, that this person would not have survived without the care of others who would educate them, support them with food and water, and promote their teachings to others. Contemporary scholarship frequently focuses premodern yoga history around an individual experience, but it is important to acknowledge that the lived reality must have been more complex and must have involved whole communities.

Although the majority of premodern yoga texts are written from the perspective of a single individual who seeks a form of liberation from their present existence, these texts must have been the work of a group of people. Consider the production of the text itself: someone must have produced the writing materials, another person dictated the text, and a scribe wrote it down.[10]

THE MAJORITY OF PREMODERN YOGA PRACTITIONERS LIVED ON THE FRINGES OF SOCIETY

For most of history, from the Vedic era to the late mediaeval period, yoga was practised only by a small number of people, predominantly located on the fringes of South Asian societies. Although some teachers, schools, and institutions enjoyed the generous patronage of local political leaders, they were not the mainstream, and many fully retreated from the society to live in the caves and woods of the Indian subcontinent. This was the case until the twentieth century, when yoga became increasingly more common, not only in India but worldwide. Today, there are yoga spaces on, figuratively speaking, every other street of Western urban areas; yet in some communities, the countercultural spirit lives on.[11]

SIX VERSES ON BECOMING TULSIDAS

Simran Uppal

Simran Uppal (they/them) is a yoga teacher, writer, and organizer based in East London. As a yoga teacher, Simran works predominantly as a faculty member for 200-hour and advanced 300-hour teacher trainings with Harriet's company: Nourish Yoga Training, an inclusive and community-oriented teacher training company based in Oxford. They've also led a wide range of continuing professional development (CPD) and public workshops in the US, across the UK, and more widely. They focus on critical approaches to the philosophical and social contexts of modern yoga, experiential and embodied forms of education, and creative, expressive movement and rest practices rooted in their own experiences of devotion, bliss, and joy in the body. They are also a community-focused organizer; most recently, they served as secretary to help found the Yoga Teachers Union UK.

As a writer, Simran has written poetry and political journalism for *The Independent*, English Heritage, and the Barbican galleries. They're also the co-director of Coriander Theatre, the UK's first theatre company made up entirely of queer people of colour. As a poet they're interested especially in radical approaches to translation from South Asian sacred texts and ecstatic poetry.

We knew Simran was the perfect choice for us to write a personal reflection on what 'honouring our sources' means in the context of being a queer, South Asian, diasporic yoga teacher and practitioner. We knew the result would be as poetic as it was political. This beautiful chapter stresses the inter-textual, interconnected, and inter-traditional nature of practice, work, and life. It centres around verses taken from the *Hanuman Chalisa*, a Hindu devotional song-poem written by Tulsidas in the sixteenth century which is today much beloved by *bhakti* practitioners and yoga teachers alike. In this chapter, Simran takes just six of the 40 dohas (verses) of the *Hanuman Chalisa*, and combines them with a mixture of translation, personal remembrances, and footnotes. This is a complex piece of work, and Simran interweaves the personal, historical, and communal in a way that demands and rewards repeated readings.

HANUMAN CHALISA, DOHA 1

shri guru charan saroj raj,   blessed guru, lotus feet dust,
nij manu mukuru sudhaari | my mind – a mirror – clear it.
barnau raghubar bimal jasu,   fruits, all four
jo daayeku phal chaari ||

From when I was small I never trusted living gurus.[i] Our gurus were alive but just in our texts, in the community itself. Later I learnt how toxic that community guru was;[ii] even later I remembered how radical it can be.[iii] The guru is in the conversation that arises between me and the text,[iv] the guru is in the spaces between, chosen family, mycelium, and roots meeting across the soil of all the world. *Mera guru*[v] is an aside from a student as they sit up from *śavāsana*, a yoga class where half the room is as queer and brown as me, the felt drawing togetherness of a murmuration in the sky.[vi]

---

i   At the gurdwara on Alice Way there are pictures showing stories of the gurus, and how now the leader of the community was the Guru Granth Sahib. I had wondered what it meant to do your *matha tek* and offer a coin before the shrine, the book the *gyani* worshipped by reading from it, white floating whisk drifting, stroked with so much meaning, above.

ii   Read Fatimah Asghar, read Ocean Vuong, read the tiredness heavy at the centre and the back of my chest, and you will know who my ancestors really are. My parents never said *lok ki kahinge?*, but only because they brought us up without Punjabi.

iii   Arvind-Pal S. Mandair, *Religion and the Specter of the West: Sikhism, India, Postcoloniality, and the Politics of Translation* (New York: Columbia University Press, 2016).

iv   I went to a lecture introducing reader response theory at uni once. I don't know who gave the lecture.

v   When Nanak was forced to work as an accountant for a wealthy landlord by his father, he got lost counting when he reached the number 13 – 10, 11, 12, *tera, tera, tera.* Thirteen but also 'yours', like 'I am yours, lover', 'I, yours, lover', yours, lover, *tera, tera, tera.* This is what authority looked like to him; born of love, not harm and use.

vi   Theodora Wildcroft, *Post-Lineage Yoga* (Sheffield: Equinox, 2020).

HANUMAN CHALISA, DOHA 2

buddhiheen tanu jaanike,
sumirau pavan-kumaar | I remember, Wind son
bal buddhi bidya dehu mohi,
harahu kales bikaar ||

Child of the winds, child of the wind-god, wind-prince. If you chant the
Chalisa through and then near the end do *jaap* of *ram*, of *sitaram*, of *sri ram
jai ram jai jai ram*, then suddenly you might feel as if you are Hanuman or
as if he is present.[i] It is not only in tantra that we instal the deity in the body.
If Rāma and Sītā are in Hanuman's heart, painted just like the sacred heart of
Jesus but with Sītā and Rāma inside, not thorns, then singing the *Chalisa* is
like finding Hanuman inside except by the end he inhabits the whole of you.[ii]

A monk at Plum Village once told a story about a little child at a *seva*
day where the monastics and laypeople were building a meditation hall
together. The monastics and laypeople (like other Buddhists they call it a
fourfold sangha, monks and nuns, men and women, but one day they will call
it something more beautiful and true) were schlepping around, carrying heavy
bricks, mixing cement, labouring heavily but probably very slowly. The little
child was just occasionally refilling a water bottle and staying out of the way
by sitting still, but turned to its parents and a monk and said, 'Ugh! No one
else does anything to help round here!' The monk looked at the child and its
very nuclear family, and realized that this was the presence of a parent inside,
as, that child.[iii] Nanak says, *pawan guru, pani pita, mata dharat mahat.*[iv]

---

i   Sivani Mata Francis, Hanuman Chalisa, from the album *Jasmine Garden* (2017), Bandcamp.

ii   In *The Bliss of Inner Fire: The Heart Practice of the Six Yogas of Naropa* (Somerville, MA: Wisdom
Publications, inc., 1998), Lama Yeshe tells you not to do a practice, because it must be done after
initiation from the right lineage teacher. Practices emerging from the top of a feudal hierarchy adopt
a feudal system of control over knowledge, control over worth. This is the book that taught me how
to experience myself as Heruka, as a vibrant body of light, as a basis for transforming the felt sense
of desire flowing round the body into blazing bliss, shooting up the spine, this bliss-wisdom of
emptiness, he calls it. The poet Annie Hayter, my housemate, calls this a 'cartography of desire'. After
I practised in this way for a few months, building to breath holding and visualization, and blazing
bliss from the root of spine through all the abdomen and thorax, I began to experience spontaneous
bliss throughout the day, sometimes so strong I felt nauseous. One day I woke up disorientated,
with bliss rippling, and stayed like that for hours until I had to run to the tiny balconette in my
room and open the doors to the freezing wind instead of throwing up everywhere. I sent my friend
Harriet a WhatsApp and she gently reeled me back in, was a teacher-friend, guided me through a
safer few months of practice.

iii It is not me who is telling this story but it could be a cloud.

iv 'The wind is my teacher; the waters are one parent and the great earth another'.

HANUMAN CHALISA, CHAUPAI 1

My friend Shreya gave me a translation, which says:

jai hanuman gyaan gun sagar |
jai kapis teehun lok ujagar ‖
ram doot atulit bal dhama |
anjani-putra pavansut nama ‖

Victory to thee, O Hanuman, Ocean of wisdom and virtue, victory to the Lord of monkeys who is well known in all the three worlds.
You, the messenger of Ram and repository of immeasurable strength, are also known as Anjaniputra and Pavanputra.[i]

I read a story about how early colonial missionaries to South Asia dropped off images of the crucifixion and statues, and pushed narratives and myths on brown people on the west coast somewhere. They all responded so happily – this person who is not only imbued with love from/for/of god but also is himself the son of some all-prevailing god – this narrative of the divine born onto earth and growing up to save us from a prevailing era of evil – this new figure popping up in a thousands of years older tradition – fab! The missionaries returned, hopeful, to find the crucifixes and various icons all happily propped up on home shrines, next to statues of baby Kṛṣna, images of Hanuman, *tat tvam asi* on palm leaf manuscripts.[ii]

HANUMAN CHALISA, CHAUPAI 2

mahabir bikram bajrangi |
kumati nivaar sumati ke sangi ‖
kanchan baran biraaj subesa |
kaanan kundal kunchit kesa ‖

---

i   The little pamphlet gives no credit or publishing information other than 'Computex Graphics / #1002 / 112 High Tech Indl. Centre, Caves Road, Jogeshwari East Mumbai 400 060. Tel: 8214386, 836 3311. Fax: 821 50004'.

ii   I don't remember where I read this story but I think I have changed it and it might not be true anyway. Reza Aslan (*Zealot: The Life and Times of Jesus of Nazareth*, London: The Westbourne Press, 2013) says the difference between history and myth is that history aims towards fact, whereas myth is concerned more about revealing truth. I don't think this binary is literally true but I do think it says something useful about the orientation of storytelling.

Hanuman is the colour of gold, how I am, not how white people who tan are.

It is hard to brush out curls to tie them into a *dastar* but once you have cracked it, oil and a wooden or sarbloh comb, a turban is the most protective hairstyle and your hair stays moisturized, happy, rich, all day.

I wonder how many people reading this have curls dark like mine, have skin gold like ours – or skin where the gold is held in richer, darker ways – and how many are reading this like hearing someone describe an album you still haven't listened to, and never really will.[i]

HANUMAN CHALISA, CHAUPAI X

tumhro mantra vibhishan maana l
lankeswar bhaye sab jag jana ll
jug sahastra jojan par bhaanu l
lilyo taahi madhur phal jaanu ll

imagine so much self-assurance you
mistake the sun for a sweet fruit, enjoy it.

Liberation is a tangerine, eaten slowly, every spray of oil from its skin met, every crackling piece of sweet citrus, flooding juice round the edges of your teeth.[ii]

Bullhe Shah says:

Deep into winter I am trapped in my house,
I search all over, find nothing.
Brahmins search through their books, look and look,
but Hari is, o Hari, pleasure-bringer, never seen.

He means that the Brahmins have trapped themselves in a house and a winter of their own making. If they could only open the door, leave behind their *pothis* inscribed with Sanskrit, throw out the vile casteism that limits them,

---

i   I had decided to give a reference to Emma Dabiri, *What White People Can Do Next: From Allyship to Coalition* (Dublin: Penguin, 2021), but really I am tired, and worried about who I am orienting this piece towards. There is no real reference for that. Translate the passage above yourself; if I taught myself to read Hindi-Urdu, Old Punjabi, Braj Bhasha, Awadhi, Digital Dictionaries of South Asia always open on the other tab, why can't you? I want to say hypocrite lecteur but that is the style of referencing I hate. I think to tell my therapist today that I am realizing always how you can't intellectualize yourself out of the emotions of oppression-based trauma, but you can do extraordinary things nonetheless.

When I return from therapy I have realized how much rock climbing, and pushing strongly, with pleasure, from the muscles deep in my glutes and hips, can help.

ii   Thich Nhat Hanh, *Tangerine meditation*

they could find a summer and a spring with warm skies and fruit wherever you look.

God has placed them in that caste, though, trapping them as much – worse – as any other. Winter in the hills in Punjab is cold. Brahminism is that for its oppressors, and a spring waiting to break for the rest. Which side do you choose to inhabit, now?[i]

HANUMAN CHALISA, CHAUPAI 39

jo yeh padhe hanuman chalisa l	Tulsidas is always a devotee of
hoye siddhi saakhi gaurisa ll	Hari.
tulsidas sada harichera l	Hanuman, stay always in my
kije naath hridaya mahn dera ll	heart.

Many genres of South and West Asian poetry have a convention where the poet signs off in the penultimate stanza or verse, naming themselves, or drawing in the memory of their name with a word that draws on its meaning. You speak out to yourself in the vocative or in apostrophes – 'o, Tulsidas, sing this song!' My name shares a root with *sumirau* in the second doha above. Nanak and the poets who came after him all used his name, as if to say that Nanak is really the one writing this poem, a parent's voice inside a child, a community body alive in each of its limbs, a light held in a series of palaces and singing out each time any devotee or person recites or sings a poem again. 'Kahai Nanak', the poems end or start: 'Nanak calls out:'. Remember this, o Tulsidas, I sing.

---

i   Jane McAlevey teaches us the heart of a political organizing conversation is to listen, listen, listen, enable anger and agency, listen, and then *ask the question*. Simply be silent, and wait.

SCIENTIFIC
ENQUIRIES INTO YOGA

6 —

THE SCIENCE OF YOGA RE-EXAMINED

Jules Mitchell

Jules Mitchell is the author of *Yoga Biomechanics: Stretching Redefined*, a unique, evidence-based exploration into the complexities of tissue mechanics and the human body's resilience and adaptability. She leads workshops and courses online and worldwide, runs a popular 300-hour yoga teacher training, frequently serves as guest faculty, and hosts a comprehensive mentoring programme to support teachers in both education and business.

Jules turned to scientific research in order to understand what was happening in yoga – as a practitioner and a yoga teacher. When people say, 'do your own research', they don't often imagine the time, money, and privilege that it takes to complete extensive training in anatomical science, nor the willingness to test every assumption in the movement lab, nor the courage to follow wherever the results take you.

Jules' work began with one question: at what point does the stretching we do in *āsana* become injurious? But as Jules shows us here, in order to understand 'what science knows' about *āsana*, we need to learn about the complex cultural framework for our bodily practices and the non-linear and multi-dimensional nature of pain. We need to unpick some nearly universal assumptions about rightness and wrongness in movement, and speculate on the moralization of postural aesthetics.

Just as all this knowledge was gathered from asking one question, so this piece, too, invites us to even further reflection on the relationship between function, performance, and injury in our practices.

In our experience and in research, the best answers are frequently those that start by unpicking a seemingly simple question.

As an educator of anatomy and biomechanics for yoga teachers, the way I talk about the body is quite different from some of my colleagues. I spend time every year in anatomy lab to inform my view, whereas another yoga educator might spend their time studying Āyurveda, somatic psychology, or body image. Each subject pertains to the physical form that we inhabit, but the lens through which we interpret and discuss this body varies. My interests lie in our tissues and their mechanical properties, the biological fabrics that we are made of and how they are affected by the tensional and compressive forces created by our movements. I've been tasked with writing a theoretical chapter, here, on what we know, and don't know, about bodies and science. As a result, this particular story leans heavily towards an *āsana* practice and its physicality.

I couldn't even begin to reduce the description of a body into a single paragraph, yet here I am attempting to do so. First and foremost, we must acknowledge that our bodies exist in a complex cultural framework influenced by authority, beliefs, education, profit, and more. Our investigation of the body, in this chapter, is in relation to how it is represented in the present-day, Western mainstream *āsana* practice. In order to assess that, I turned to a comprehensive survey conducted in the US that reported the majority of both practising and non-practising adults view yoga mostly as for the body, to improve flexibility, and that it is ultimately 'good for you'.[1] In light of these results, the narrative within this chapter will focus on how an individual body appears, functions, and feels through the lens of teaching yoga.

Science, as a system, is more about getting closer to the truth than it is about proving an absolute truth. Data are often misinterpreted and sometimes weaponized to make overreaching conclusions, usually to the support or discredit of certain stakeholders. Science, especially as it relates to biology, cannot possibly distinguish right from wrong, fact from fiction, or even truth from fallacy. It is better suited as a system that helps us weigh benefits versus risks or determine a relatively reliable course of action. Research in the field of exercise science and rehabilitation rarely solves a single problem with a single, clear intervention. In practice, out in the world outside of the biomechanics lab, the pursuit of knowledge requires that we balance empiricism with data. Because science exists within the same social, political, economic, and epistemological frameworks in which our bodies also exist, its interpretation is subject to one's lived experience. Spend enough time in the world of research and academia, and you will discover that the context of experiments influences their conclusions. One study may report on injuries within yoga and raise concerns surrounding the safety of the practice. Another study may report on injuries across a variety of physical activities, absolving concerns about yoga's safety in comparison to rugby or American football. The relative occurrence of yoga related adverse events in each study could be identical, but the surrounding context tells quite a different story, influencing the interpretation. Science, therefore, is best applied to mainstream yoga as a tool to guide you to ask more nuanced questions than you have before; a method by which you begin to discern what you learned in your yoga teacher training and what you want your future continuing education to include.

Finally, how am I defining mainstream yoga? Loosely, I'm referring to the practice as it has been shared and popularly consumed in the West over the last 50 years. More specifically, I'm focusing on how we teach modern postural yoga (MPY) as a result of the rising popularity of yoga teacher training schools over the last 20 years. The intention of this chapter is to expose what we know about bodies and science *today*, and I believe the trends of the last two decades make an excellent theoretical model to explore what we think we know versus what we know. Additionally, as I'm an exercise scientist, not a historian, nor a sociologist, I will leave the history and analysis of the term MPY to the appropriate experts. My use of the term is to refer to a specific aspect of the vastly larger practice that yoga defines, not to scrutinize the emergence or implications of the term. I acknowledge the controlled boundaries I have created here, and consequently encourage you, the reader, to layer on for yourself any additional perspectives pertaining to your own areas of expertise and personal experience.

Let's return now to how the body appears, functions, and feels, and how yoga is viewed as a practice that improves upon these measures. We know the body is a highly adaptable structure that can improve or decline, with tissues that can synthesize or degrade, and has experiences that can be positive or negative. Yoga is one avenue for the pursuit of physical improvements, but it certainly is not the only avenue. In my years of studying and teaching biomechanics and yoga, two other topics captured my attention: posture and flexibility. The published scientific literature on these two topics is more abundant than it is on yoga (although recent years suggest that won't always be the case), making posture and flexibility excellent comparisons for the discussion at hand. You'll discover that the evolution of MPY in the West follows a surprisingly predictable path. You've heard the phrase 'history repeats itself'? We might also say that *society repeats itself*, especially in how we measure positive effects on the body and how we frame the validity of the measurements themselves.

APPEARANCE, AESTHETICS, AND STATURE

An observation I often share about yoga is how different it is than just about any other exercise or movement modality because *you're not actually moving*. Of course, you're moving to get from one pose to the next, but these movements are discussed separately from the poses and are even described as the 'transitions' between the postures. The transitions rarely get any attention in most styles of MPY, and when they do, they are usually measured in terms of creativity rather than technique. Yoga, after all, is not a competitive sport where enhanced technique results in a winner; the transition is not about getting you into the pose faster or hitting your mark with more accuracy. Instead, yoga poses are instructed by their appearance (e.g. in Triangle Pose, you organize your limbs into a series of triangles).

The aesthetic nature of the static yoga pose lends itself perfectly to an evaluation based on 'alignment'. Essentially each pose, or even more appropriately named, *posture*, is satisfied by a specific arrangement of parts. These anatomical parts, observed at the gross anatomical level, resemble a series of lines (long bones), and their angles of connection (joints). Since lines and angles make up shapes (not the same as getting 'in shape' but also not a 'stretch' in the current discussion), it is easy to extrapolate basic geometry lessons, mainly perpendicular lines that form right angles, into alignment-based teaching. Unfortunately, the rules of Euclidean geometry that we learned in school apply to a very specific set of conditions, which biology does not inhabit.[i] When we teach Warrior One Pose with a specific angle to create with the ankle, knee, and hip, and the arms reaching overhead in a parallel arrangement we are projecting a system that works best with pen and paper onto our anatomy, not actually expressing any biomechanical measure. This doesn't make the angles and the lines we use to assess yoga poses *wrong*; but it is reductionist.

We can, in fact, explore biomechanical data on various alignments in a static pose with the use of technology. Recently, a paper examined the biomechanics of Triangle Pose in three different stance lengths and found that

---

i   There are entirely different systems of geometry (i.e. fractal, spherical, hyperbolic) which have entirely different sets of rules, but unless you specialize in mathematics or a related field, you'll probably never learn about them.

in the frontal plane the longest stance increased load on the front ankle, knee, and hip and decreased the load on the back ankle, and knee.[2] As someone who has spent considerable time in a biomechanics lab and studying free body diagrams, the results were intuitive to me as the head, trunk, and pelvis are all leaning away from the base of support of the back leg, but I would not expect yoga teachers to make the same assumption, particularly when sensation might tell a different story. Again, this is not a criticism of MPY nor its teachers, rather an exploration of how aesthetics leads us to believe we know something (longer stance alignment is harder or more advanced) different than what is true (in this case, the longer stance is easier on the back knee and ankle).

To complicate matters further, the calculations used to derive the data in these yoga studies are also based in Euclidean geometry, as well as Newtonian physics. We know our musculoskeletal tissues are viscoelastic,[i] and thereby exhibit non-Newtonian behaviour. Do you see the conflict? We are applying models that do not fit and then forming conclusions based on the ill-fitting outcomes. Until we can apply a more appropriate model, however, we must work with what we have. Classical biomechanics studies, in conjunction with fields of study such as tissue mechanics and biotensegrity,[ii] can provide richer layers of interpretation and help prevent overly simplistic conclusions.

Speaking of overly simplistic conclusions, one of the most offensive conclusions I have come across is that there is a single correct shape or alignment for a static yoga pose. While it may seem obvious to everyone that there is not, a growing trend using artificial intelligence to 'evaluate how well a pose is performed' suggests otherwise.[3] As a technology enthusiast, the implementation of computer-based learning to instruct yoga poses is attractive. As a biomechanist, the implementation of computer-based pose recognition and grading is concerning. Any system that values the poses on *what they look like* will only tether us tighter to the alignment framework. The leap from 'being in good shape' to 'being in *a* good shape' is already too short in MPY and we should employ technologies that promote autonomy and self-assessment over external correctives.

We already struggle with visually assessing yoga poses based on beliefs regarding safety. On one hand we are told certain shapes are risky: deep backbends are called out as careless, extreme flexibility becomes irresponsible, and certain postures are identified as ones to avoid altogether. In this narrative, yoga, which the general public tends to view as 'for the body' and 'good for

---

i   Exhibiting both viscous and elastic properties; time-dependent relationship to stress and strain.
ii   Application of tensegrity principles to biological systems.

you' now becomes an exercise of restraint; do less, hold back, and even, avoid. On the other hand, we are told certain shapes are healing: backbends correct our rounded postures, flexibility keeps us young and supple, certain postures have (albeit overstated) physiological benefits. In this narrative, yoga now becomes an exercise of unconstraint; do more, go for it, and even, push through. The messaging is confusing at best but does the most harm by disempowering teachers who are led to rely on what they see.

Returning to biomechanical studies, what I find problematic about most of them is the assumption that lower loads are safer than higher loads, even when there are no adverse events in the subjects. Comparative data suggest that the forces in yoga are similar to other non-risky fitness activities that healthy populations engage in regularly.[4] For example, we know that the ground reaction force (GRF)[i] in running is roughly twice that of slow walking. From that, we do not conclude that running should be avoided. Similarly, pose variations with higher loads do not need to be avoided simply because of the load. In fact, the evidence tells us that yoga is generally safe and the occurrences of adverse incidents are similar to 'physical activity and usual care'.[5] The interpretation and application of these data do, however, exist in the complex framework mentioned previously and will be influenced by the teacher's world view.

It's important to note here that the debates around the shape of the body are not exclusive to yoga. It is a common theme in sports and rehab as well. You've likely engaged in the recent debate regarding the knee angle in a squat. Thirty years ago, the National Strength and Conditioning Association (NSCA) published a position statement on the squat, mainly in regard to the knee joint and spine, citing the relevant literature at the time. It suggested that both structures were generally safe in a loaded squat although some squatting forms were riskier than others.[6] This is an example of a scientific statement where the intention is to get closer to the truth instead of proving a point. Something can be generally safe yet impose a small-level risk, such as driving a car, taking most medications, even practising yoga! Yet a statement such as the NCSA position requires a depth of understanding in the topic at hand to tease out the nuance. Most trainers and coaches who don't specialize in squat biomechanics miss that depth and thus debate good form versus bad form in the absence of necessary caveats. When driving a car or taking medications, widespread social acceptance and clear benefits make it easier to accept any

---

i   A ground reaction force is the force exerted by the earth onto a body contacting it. At rest (e.g. Mountain Pose) the GRF corresponds to your body weight. As you move, acceleration increases, therefore GRF increases.

risk of harm. In the case of yoga, widespread social acceptance for the last 50 years has recently shifted from an overall panacea to body wrecker.[7] This polarized debate calls for a more nuanced conversation.

This conundrum is not new. In fact, it's played out almost exactly like this in the realms of posture and flexibility. Bodily posture is much like a specific yoga posture in that it is judged by how it appears. Good posture is generally accepted as better for you. It's easy to see why we think correct yoga alignment is also better for you. Flexibility is also judged by how it appears. The internet will tell you if you can't touch your toes, you're in bad shape. It's easy to see why we collapse the shape of a yoga pose with being *in* shape. A bit of history on the social acceptance around posture and flexibility over the years could serve us quite well in the MPY conversation.

Let's start with posture. Have you ever been told to sit up straight by a parent or schoolteacher? Or had a non-industry friend comment on your form when engaging in a household task? These well-meaning comments are rooted in a long and fascinating history of posture and what is *considered* proper. I emphasize *considered* because proper depends on the trends of a particular era. Several hundred years ago in Europe, slouching was a luxury afforded by the aristocrats. Meanwhile, the military was establishing an ideal weapon-wielding posture that evolved into the discipline-demonstrating posture of an effective soldier. This ultimately entered the mainstream as a stature-flaunting posture. Social elites were sold on stiffer postures and behaviours. This became an easily identifiable visual criterion for judging good versus bad. During the end of the nineteenth century and beginning of the twentieth century good posture became an indicator for health and wellness, as well as morals and status, amplified by the medicalization, and subsequently the monetization of posture.[8] If capitalism can create a problem, it can also sell you a solution, especially as it pertains to the body. Eventually, more casual postures returned during the mid-twentieth century, but capitalism keeps the good versus bad debate thriving. Today, MPY follows a similar path where good yoga alignment represents a skilled and dedicated practitioner and, in many spheres, is still considered a superior way of practising.

A similar story is true for flexibility and range of motion (ROM). Have you ever heard someone say they should stretch more? Has someone explained they can't participate in a certain activity because they don't have enough flexibility? These misguided comments are similarly rooted in fluctuating trends embraced by society, also with an interesting history. People have been stretching for millennia, mostly likely because it just feels good. Yet, certain cultures during certain eras seem to have also stretched to improve or prepare the body to get in shape for specific activities, including military activities. About one hundred years ago, the mainstream adopted stretching through various calisthenic and gymnastic-type practices.[9] Eventually, the American College of Sports Medicine (ACSM) named flexibility as one of the five components of fitness and ROM became an official measure for being in shape.[10] While flexibility didn't quite stretch to indicate morality, having limited ROM implied a less than optimal physicality. The research community has aggressively challenged this notion in the last 20 years, unsuccessfully trying to invalidate stretching recommendations.[11] This helps explain the present-day divide around flexibility. On one hand, industry professionals familiar with the research maintain that flexibility does not matter as much as society believes it does. On the other hand, non-industry people are known for guiltily confessing that they don't stretch enough. MPY follows a similar divide where for some people, yoga is a flexibility exercise and for others, yoga's emphasis on flexibility is its problem.

To summarize, assessing and teaching yoga postures based on the way they appear has limited value. Yes, you could quickly sketch a mathematical model in your head to guess where loads might be higher or lower, but it won't tell you what the person in the pose can withstand nor what they feel. Additionally, what we say about the aesthetics of a pose is part of a larger social framework. As these ideas are disseminated into the yoga community, definitions of alignment are changing. Those once branded as alignment teachers are subtly changing their language to say things such as *inner* alignment, *individual* alignment, and 'aligned with your intention'. It's a clever and necessary way to avoid a total rebrand, protect your customer base, and circumvent a formal declaration that your teaching is changing now that certain beliefs are falling out of fashion. As the cultural landscape shifts, so must the business model. And this is exactly why we, as a society, will always struggle to separate what science says from how science is interpreted.

FUNCTION, PERFORMANCE, AND INJURY

Another observation I share about MPY is how often we cue the pose *after we are already in the pose*. Of course, since the static shape is the focus, and the transitions are relatively quick, the time to talk about the pose is in the pose. Sometimes those cues encourage observations and experiences, and other times those cues imply correcting and protecting. The latter leads to a perception that yoga, and more specifically, properly instructed yoga, leads to improvements in how the body performs.

The static nature of yoga poses might place them in a category of exercises called isometrics, where muscles engage yet remain the same length, maintaining a static joint position. However, remaining still, or not moving, does not automatically imply the muscles are overcoming any substantial resistance that would result in favourable adaptations to biomotor abilities such as strength or endurance. [i] One of the most basic biomechanics principles, progressive overload, explains how increasing any number of load parameters is essential to promote increases in tissue capacity. It is certainly possible that some poses meet these requirements in some individuals, but as a general rule most do not (e.g. in Tree Pose the knee extensor joint moment of force[ii] in the sagittal plane of the standing leg is a fraction of what it is during a casual walking pace).[12]

The SAID principle (specific adaptations to imposed demands)[iii] reminds us that improving a particular skill or generating a physiological adaptation requires a specific set of inputs. Consider the physical demands and load parameters of yoga, and you'll discover they closely resemble a static stretching routine or mobility programme. Not surprisingly, yoga helps with flexibility. The ACSM, however, classifies yoga as neuromotor fitness, placing the biomotor abilities of balance and coordination in the foreground. Naturally, flexibility and balance will carry over a small amount to the overall function of the body, but not enough to be considered specific training. Consequently, the research on the impact of both flexibility and yoga on various metrics of physical performance is vast, exhaustive, and underwhelmingly benign.

This news should be a welcome relief. Yoga teachers need not take on the responsibility of training biomotor abilities that are not inherently part of the practice. Yoga doesn't have to make you stronger, faster, or more powerful. Yoga might make you more flexible, but it doesn't have to do that either. Yoga can simply improve your mind/body connection and any other abilities that carry over too. This includes the vague promise of becoming more functional.

Functional movement is mostly a marketing term, as any movement you do is functional if you want to move that way. Injuries are probably the only thing we can all agree are not functional. Injured bodies don't perform

---

i   Biomotor abilities are skills/functions related to physical performance such as agility, coordination, speed, mobility, etc.

ii   Joint moments of force are the product of the magnitude and distance from the reference joint to where the load is applied.

iii The SAID principle explains that the human body under biomechanical or neurological stress will adapt specifically to the type of stress, with minimal carry-over. For example, playing the piano might make learning the guitar easier because you can read sheet music, but you still need to specifically practise playing the guitar. Likewise, cycling may improve your cardiovascular endurance, but if you plan to run a marathon, you should specifically train for long-distance running.

well, and injured tissues don't transmit force well, impairing their primary function. This brings up the complicated matter of cueing corrections and protections while already in the pose. Can we, with any certainty, know that the micro-movements and minor joint adjustments are having a functional effect, especially since the function to get into the pose was already there? We know that yoga is overwhelmingly safe despite very little standardization of how it's taught and what cues are offered.[13] Knowing this, and a little tissue mechanics, should help give confidence to teachers.

Tissue mechanics is the study of the mechanical properties of biological materials. In exercise science, these tissues are mostly musculoskeletal, including muscles and collagen-based structures like bones, cartilage, tendons, and ligaments. These collagen tissues absorb and transmit tensional and compressive forces, and have so many fascinating features they could fill a textbook. Collagen has such immense tensile strength; it's often compared to a steel cable. These tissues are highly resistant to acute injuries and the more you load them, the more resistant they become (think of building bone density with weight-bearing exercises). The rate and magnitude of load that causes an injury are extremely high (think of breaking a bone because of a fall). Think of the typical loads present in yoga poses and compare them to other activities with high injury risks and you'll recognize that yoga has a relatively low injury risk but might not prevent injuries in sports where the loads are faster and higher. Unfortunately, injury is yet another area that exists in our complex cultural framework. Definitions are regulated, and diagnoses are part of medical treatments belonging to a hierarchical medical system. This makes talking about injuries and injury prevention a very loaded topic.

The expectation that yoga poses improve aspects of physicality, including performance and function, follows a similar path to the posture and flexibility stories. Good posture was aesthetically pleasing, but also reflected a body well constructed and free from deformity, and signalled optimal physical functioning.[14] Since MPY is entangled with posture culture, it's easy to believe that well-taught, properly instructed, poses can avoid injury, despite no evidence to suggest that. Stretching improves the ranges in which you move and is also believed to enhance performance and prevent injury. Since yoga is so heavily associated with flexibility, it's easy to see why society collapses the effects of stretching onto yoga. Yet research into stretching tells us those beliefs are just beliefs. After decades of research, a systematic review by an extremely well-respected team tells us stretching right before an activity yields small detriments in performance and mostly doesn't prevent injury.[15] Subsequent publications consider flexibility exercises a useful component in most warm-up routines when combined with other *sport-specific* selections.[16] In summary, a routine yoga practice will probably improve your yoga practice more than any other measure of function or performance.

SENSATION, DISCOMFORT, AND PAIN

A final observation I share about MPY is how much the teachers care about the students. Regardless of the style of yoga they teach, what got them into teaching yoga, or which side of the alignment/safety fence they sit on, they all agree they want their students to have a yoga experience that is delightful and pain free. It's a fortunate agreement because that is really all we can offer. As you can see, much of what we believe about teaching yoga is influenced by far more than what science tells us. Science is better at telling us what we are getting wrong, not what is right. That doesn't mean you should give up on your education.

A commitment to the study of biomechanics inevitably leads to the study of pain science. Tissue mechanics shows us the body is a highly adaptable structure that can improve or decline, with tissues that can synthesize or degrade, but it does not explain why things hurt. Posture research reveals that good posture does not equal pain free. Stretching studies tell us that improvements in range of motion have little to do with changes in tissue length and more to do with how someone tolerates the sensation of the stretch. The yoga literature casts a wide net over the various physiological and psychological conditions it can positively affect but isn't able to identify which feature of the yoga is the active ingredient. Pain science, however, explains why different people feel different things in different poses.

Biology is complicated, so is pain. Both are non-linear and multi-dimensional, meaning they are hard to quantify. For example, consider the relationship between tissue damage and pain. If these two variables had a linear relationship each unit of tissue damage would result in an additional unit of pain. A paper cut would mean very little pain and a rotator cuff tear would mean much more pain. Yet plenty of people have asymptomatic rotator cuff tears but a paper cut with a little lemon juice would likely bring them to their knees. Another example is osteoarthritis (OA). People with OA tend to have good days and bad days. If the relationship between OA and pain were linear, the cartilage would be regenerating on good days and degrading on bad days, but that is not the case. These two-dimensional models do not account for other variables that are inherent to our lived experience such as sleep, nutrition, disease, trauma, stress, and belief.

What does this mean for teaching yoga? It means you can't look at someone in the pose and know if they are in pain. It means you can't cue a more functional joint position and know it won't cause them pain. I find this realization to be quite liberating for yoga teachers. Instead of protecting and correcting you can guide the experience of the pose. If you want to teach Triangle Pose as a series of triangles, you can; and they don't have to be perfect Euclidean triangles. You can choose action cues such as push, reach, pull, or press over positional or postural cues. Most MPY teachers already have an arsenal of these cues, thus it often becomes a matter of simply saying a little less. That extra space leaves opportunities to guide autonomy and self-assessment.

I frequently hear that yoga teachers should teach students the difference between pain and discomfort. I agree with the sentiment but disagree with the implementation. Pain is subjective and, as we now know, non-linear and multi-dimensional. No person can explain to another what pain feels like or what discomfort feels like. They're as hard to describe as water. Moreover, some people thrive in discomfort while others will have a debilitating flare-up for the three days following. Only the individual can distinguish the difference for themselves, which is where yoga teachers can have a profound impact. By framing the postures as opportunities to observe and experience various sensations, as well as the effects of them in the following days, the teacher can shift the responsibility back to the student, which is where it ultimately belongs.

We could draw similar parallels in the posture and flexibility realms. We can't look at someone with poor posture and assume they hurt. Likewise, we can't assume that fixing someone's posture when they are in pain will alleviate their pain. We can certainly suggest a change in posture and empirically test if they notice a change. If they do, we can't extrapolate that same result to the population at large. Of course, it's easier to accept this now that we've explored the cultural paradigm in which posture exists.[17] Fixing poor posture is an easy sell: far easier than the uncertainty I've created here. The same is true for flexibility. We can't assume someone with a limited range of motion has poor physical function or is in pain. In fact, when we see tight students struggle, shake, and grunt, it's usually when we are instructing them to push into the limits of their range. They probably aren't affected during their morning jog or evening stroll. Once again, our beliefs about flexibility, and the meaning we make, are rarely in line with what science tells us.

In conclusion, we know a lot about the body, yet we know very little about the body. We know it's robust and resilient and has the capacity to become more so. Whether yoga can, or should, increase that capacity is still under scrutiny. We now understand that social beliefs around posture and flexibility are heavily reflected in MPY, and we can look to research in all three areas to start to build a new narrative. Near the beginning of the chapter, I proposed that just as history repeats itself, *society repeats itself.* The good news is that we can learn from the past and we can learn from our communities. I invite you to share what you've learned here with your own yoga communities so we can start to build a new narrative informed by science.

7

ENQUIRY AND INTENTION IN THE TEACHING OF YOGA

Peter Blackaby

Peter Blackaby has been teaching yoga since 1986. He is an anatomy specialist, who is also trained in osteopathy. For the past 15 years his central interest has been the development of his humanistic yoga courses, which aim to integrate modern understandings of neurology, psychology, and biomechanics into yoga. His work is an accessible and understated case study in how to bridge both somatic and scientific approaches to movement.

In this piece, Peter explores the relationship between intention and attention, using this to differentiate between exercise, performance, and yoga, and encouraging us to understand the unique place that yoga holds in this typology. With that understanding, he carefully explores the ambient, conditioned, and traumatic reasons for our movement habits, and how these affect the meaning we find in the world around us. But he also offers a set of questions for framing practice that work to build somatic awareness, questions that we can use both in our own practice, and with others.

Like Peter, we believe a somatic approach is one of the most effective ways to integrate contemporary scientific understandings into a traditional yogic approach of self-discovery and self-awareness. In our experience, while many yoga teachers are intrigued by somatic styles of movement, few have been given the skills to teach others in this kind of experiential exploration. And yet, teachers exploring similar approaches, including many of the other teachers in this book, are often highly respected, but rarely famous. They are the 'expert's experts' of yoga teaching.

Teaching by rote instruction is easier, more popular with beginners and casual practitioners, and is the natural expression of a view of bodies and science that is universalized and standardized. But once we start to understand that real life, real bodies, and real science are a lot more complicated than that, it is time to embrace a more complex pedagogy, with more cautious answers to offer.

Yoga is a broad church with a long and rich history, and, like much of Indian thinking, it seamlessly weaves together both religious and philosophical thought. This can be perplexing for the Western mind, which tends to separate out theology from philosophy. What is clear, though, is that, at its heart, yoga is a soteriology, offering liberation from suffering. To be clear, this does not mean the *avoidance* of suffering. It means fully engaging in all aspects of life and meeting whatever life brings with attention and curiosity, however difficult the subject – because there is no doubt that a life well lived will bring many challenges. My interest and my perspective as a man brought up in a Western culture is how to practise and teach yoga in a way that stays true to its aims of reducing suffering but is also situated in the here and now, in the world I inhabit.

One of the most compelling ideas that has arisen in the last couple of hundred years is that of evolution. There are still plenty of unanswered questions, both cosmological and biological, but most of us would be very surprised to find out that this theory was wildly wrong. It is the most likely explanation of how life emerged in the starkness of the universe. The animation of matter, or how chemistry became biology, is particularly mysterious. Life emerged from matter...yet it never became apart from matter, and one of the most extraordinary aspects of living things is their ability to maintain their physical integrity in a changing world. This process is called homeostasis. In simple organisms this is regulated through the membrane of a cell or cells, excreting harmful molecules through the membrane and absorbing those it needs. In complex creatures like human beings, elaborate mechanisms evolved to keep critical aspects of physiology within the bounds necessary to maintain life and all this regulation goes on at an autonomic level. We are unaware of these processes unless they become dis-regulated for some reason, and when this happens it is brought to our attention via our sensory nervous system with increasing urgency. Anyone who has swum underwater will know this: the longer you are underwater the more compelling the urge to breathe becomes. Our sensory nervous system is the tool we have to alert us to suffering when our body moves away from homeostasis but it isn't limited to yoga. Dis-regulation of our social world is flagged up by another group of sensations we label as emotions or mood. How comfortable or uncomfortable we feel in our community will be noticed as various feelings of well-being and distress. If we see examples of unfairness at play in our community, we feel a sense of anger or outrage. When we notice acts of kindness and compassion, we feel a sense of gratitude and warmth. The point of course is that these feelings motivate behaviour in a direction of social homeostasis in an attempt to reduce suffering and enhance flourishing.

Clearly then, being interested in what our body is trying to tell us with sensation, feelings, and moods is far more likely to bring about a life that harmonizes with its environment and those around us.

Each part of the sensory nervous system plays a part in life maintenance, which I will briefly review here.

THE NERVOUS SYSTEM

Simply put, there is a world out there that we notice with our sensory nervous system. We make sense of what we notice in our brain and we respond to what we notice through our motor system. It is worth thinking a bit more about the nature of the sensory part of our nervous systems, which we could describe in five main parts:

1. Our *exteroceptors* inform us about the outside world via sight, sound, smell, temperature, balance, touch, and to some extent pain. When we consider why these senses evolved, it is obvious that it was to help keep us safe in a dangerous and unpredictable world. The more we can notice the world and recognize danger and where safety lies, the longer we are liable to survive.

2. Our *interoceptors* inform us about our internal environment through sensations from our viscera. They let us know when we are hungry or thirsty, or when we need to go to the toilet. They regulate our breathing, as well as any uncomfortable feelings in our stomach, and so on. The point here, of course, is to keep our internal world safe and within defined homeostatic boundaries. Ignoring these feelings risks the deregulation of our internal environment.

3. Our *proprioceptors* inform us about how our body is navigating the world we inhabit. They tell us where our body is positioned in space, how fast it is moving, and how much effort it is exerting. Ignoring these sensations can lead to awkward movements, over-stretching, and injury when lifting or moving things around.

4. *Nociceptors* are nerve endings found in the skin, mucosa, muscles, joints, and much of the viscera and digestive tract of the body. They respond to damage in neighbouring tissue and let the brain know anything that might be of concern to the organism. Whether nociception is experienced as pain will depend on many things, such as whether similar experiences have been felt before, and how much the person worries about the sensation. In other words, nociception is highly modifiable by the context of the situation. A feeling of discomfort will be amplified by someone who is worried by the sensation, and down-modulated by someone who does not feel so worried about the feeling.

5. Non-sensory input can come from other regions of the brain, and includes memories, beliefs, and expectations. All other forms of sensory input will be, to a greater or lesser extent, modified by our prior experience. Surprisingly, even sight is modified by experience. If you doubt this, Google 'Adelson's Checker-Shadow Illusion' and you will find that what we see is really what we expect to see.

The point about this brief foray into the sensory nervous system is to recognize that it exists to keep us safe, to guide us through an unpredictable world. Anything potentially harmful will either have been seen or felt as discomfort. If we ignore these signals, it is likely they will get louder until we take notice and either reflect on or modify our behaviour. Yoga, as I see it, is explicitly about our ability to notice how and what we feel, reflect on that perception, and then act in a way that reduces harm to you and those around you. It is in this way we reduce suffering. However, we also have to be mindful of the nature of the brain and the way it is set up to see, feel, and generally sense what it expects – and expectation will be largely determined by the culture and individual history of the person involved. I would like to argue that the point of yoga, which also keeps it close to its soteriological roots, is to examine closely what it is we actually notice, what it means to us, and how we are going to respond to it. I would like to differentiate this from *intention* in exercise and performance. Both exercise and performance are often considered aspects of yoga, but in my view their starting points – their different intentions – make them something different.

EXERCISE

The intention of exercise is to change structure: to become stronger, more flexible, or more aerobically fit. It is intention that is the designating factor. Mowing the lawn can be considered exercise, but I am going to call that 'activity', as the *intention* is to mow the lawn – any effect on structure is a happy side effect. If I go to the gym and lift weights or step on a running machine, my concern is to *exercise* my muscles or cardiovascular system. Exercise follows two biological laws, Wolff's and Davis's. Wolff's law states that bones will adapt their strength according to the load imposed on them, both in the trabecular and cortical parts of the bone.[1] Davis's law says similar things about soft-tissue remodelling – the more familiar idea that muscles, tendons, ligaments, and associated fascia also enlarge under load and diminish when rested over an extended period of time.[2] For structure to change, load is imperative but attention is not. In its most basic form, a muscle can have its strength maintained by regular electrical stimulation. A person could be in a coma, yet his or her muscles can be prevented from atrophy by regular electrical stimulation. These muscles, though, are not developing 'intelligence'. There is no environment they are responding to. It is in a sense the 'stupidest' form of exercise, although a necessity in those who through some misfortune are unable to contract their own muscles. In a gym, muscles can be toned in many ways, using body weight, resistance machines or bands, or by lifting free weights. Depending on what you are doing, attention is only partially required – it is quite possible to do a workout listening to your favourite music, with only scant attention paid to what you are doing. It is true, of course, that some exercises can be made trickier and draw our attention in, but now attention is the happy by-product of exercise, the changing of structure. Many people enjoy and derive pleasure from exercise, of course. There can be psychological uplifts from the sense of agency or feeling of virtuousness that someone feels when doing something for their health. And exercise often combines with friendship to engender a sense of fraternity. These things can be part of the way we maintain a sense of well-being, but they are not a soteriology – an enquiry into ourselves with a purpose of reducing suffering and promoting flourishing.

PERFORMANCE

The intention of performance is to achieve something, and often to perfect something. It could be anything from a strenuous gymnastics display or dance piece to the playing of a piece of music. Structure is much less important here, although the gymnast will be working seriously on their structure while going through their routine. Structure is the means to serve an end, which is the performance. Two things are essential in improving a performance: we must repeat what we are doing many hundreds or thousands of times; and, while repeating the movements, we must pay attention to how and what we are doing, with the intention of improving. In this there is certainly some overlap with yoga. The focused attention that is required brings the performer into the moment – past and future evaporate under the attention required to hone a performance. Second, in performance, one's physical sense of well-being may be sacrificed for the sake of the art. Stories of ballerinas dancing on broken toes are a good example. The direction of attention is not on the discrimination of perception, rather it is the overriding of it in the pursuit of excellence. In other words, when the goal becomes the object, it is often at the cost of how we feel. In yoga classes, too, people often try to push themselves to achieve a particular shape because the shape is seen as the primary concern, with sensation secondary.

I have intentionally drawn lines here between what could be called exercise, performance, and yoga. In life, of course, these lines are blurred and elements of all three are generally present, but clarifying these distinctions can help us orientate our practice or our teaching.

YOGA

Yoga, I am arguing, has its intention rooted in the notion that we want to reduce suffering, both in ourselves and in the world we inhabit. The tools we have are those that evolved under evolutionary pressure: a sensory nervous system that informs us about the outside world, our inside world and the tissues of our body, and a brain and body that perceive these sensations and give them meaning, on which we act. *How* we act gives rise to feelings and emotions that feel good or not so good, and it is these feelings that guide our trajectory through life. If only it were so simple... The problem is that perception can be and often is distorted by culture and individual history. We form habits, biases, and beliefs on our journey through life.

HABITS, BIASES, AND BELIEFS

As noted earlier, perception of sensation is always coloured by the expectations that history places on it. In fact, perception seems to be predictive: our brain predicts what it notices, based on what it has noticed before. Our world of experience is not an accurate read of the world as it is, rather a montage of sensations given meaning by a brain that constantly tries to present a coherent and meaningful picture of the world to the organism it is part of. We learn both movement and behaviour as maps of action in response to the events we notice sensorially. One way of thinking about this is to categorize our habits, biases, and beliefs about the world into three main groups: those that are ambient; those that are conditioned; and those that are traumatically embedded.

Ambient habits

These are the habits of body and behaviour that we breathe in by osmosis, simply by existing in a particular culture at a particular time. Bodily, we may start to stand, sit, or walk like those we grow up around – our family or peers will exert a gentle shaping of body and mind simply because of the waters we swim in, much like the way a prevailing wind will shape the way the branches of a tree grow. Your family may walk, swim, or cycle as their form of recreation or do nothing at all. A family might be boisterous, untidy, and spontaneous or they may be organized and tidy with a tendency to plan everything. These things will feel normal to the child growing up in such environments. No value judgement is placed on it, it is just normal life. Ambient habits are what we do to fit in with our surroundings. We generally do not even notice ambient habits until we leave home and meet other people who grew up in different households with different ambient habits. This can be both an exciting and an anxious time, full of new and unfamiliar ideas and different ways of seeing the world. We may lose some of the habits we grew up with and adopt or form new ones that help us fit comfortably into our new environment. If, however, this does not happen, an ambient habit may start to ossify – our constant shifting of weight to one side may in the end make it impossible to shift the weight to the other side. Once this happens, a bias becomes a constraint and our life loses choice. If we stay within one family or community, our psychological habits may start to become bigoted. Our views of the world stay narrow, never challenged, and again they become a constraint.

Conditioned habits (beliefs)

These are habits that have a value imposed on them in the body. When we are told to sit up straight or stand up straight, we are told so because culturally these postures are perceived to be morally superior to less upright ones. These ideas about how to 'hold' the body permeate the military, ballet, yoga, and schools of deportment, but the trouble is once we start to behave in a particular way at the expense of our feelings, we begin the process of fragmentation between sensation and response. Slumping is a normal response to tiredness, and movement a natural response to feelings of stiffness, so asking a child to sit still and sit up straight is asking them to believe that how you look is more important than how you feel. If this process continues throughout life, we may lose the ability to know how we are really feeling and how to respond to those feelings. We do not notice until we are in pain. That pain can then seem mysterious, appearing out of nowhere with no apparent reason. This is also true of psychological beliefs, habits, and biases that are given a moral value. When we are told something is right by an authority figure but feel it is wrong inside, discomfort of some sort is nearly always the result. This may manifest as anxiety or depression, but equally it could appear as headaches, stomach upsets, or musculoskeletal pain.

Traumatic habits

When something overwhelms our ability to respond appropriately, our body will often respond automatically. We might engage our fight/flight responses, we might freeze, or even fall asleep. These responses are beyond our control – they seem to happen *to* us. The initial cause of these responses may also become triggering events in the future. When I was in my thirties, I was involved in a serious road accident, and the piece of music that was playing in my car at the moment of impact still causes a lurch in my stomach and feeling of worry when I hear it, until I recognize what is happening. More serious traumas when triggered can cause feelings of paralysis or dissociation, and dis-enable a person in such a way that they are unable to function normally in life.

Whether habits are ambient, conditioned, or traumatic, they are all unconscious responses to life events that may interfere with a person's ability to have choice about the way they live their lives and, as such, there is great value in investigating them further. It is important to stress that the formation of habits and biases is an intelligent response to the situation that formed the person. It is not some sort of malfunction. It is also important to recognize that most of our habits serve us very well and all that is needed is to keep them functioning efficiently for us. Problems occur because we and the world that we inhabit are in a constant state of change. A habit formed in one situation may not serve a person when they are older and the world has changed. When this happens, we tend to suffer in one form or another because our habits have become a constraint.

There is another interesting aspect to habits that needs consideration, which is that, no matter how much we repeat them, we do not change them – they normally stay the same, with no new learning taking place. Moshé Feldenkrais once made this point about handwriting, asking the question 'Whose handwriting is perfect?' The answer of course is hardly anyone's, and this is true of almost any motor function or behaviour in life: we learn to do something until it serves our purpose and then the performance plateaus out. If we want to make further progress we need to repeat what we are doing with a clear intention of improving what we are doing. This is the process of adaptation – our behaviour changes skilfully to meet our new situation more comfortably, and as we do this we suffer less.

Practice

Even the most comfortable life will imprint itself on a growing person. As noted previously, ambient habits will ease into a life by osmosis. Beliefs will settle into our unconscious and everyday worries and anxieties will tend to tighten us in our own particular ways. If we are lucky, these things will shape us positively, becoming the characteristics we are then known by – the way we move, the things we laugh at, our energy (or lack of it) become the grounds on which our lives are writ. If we are less lucky, these habits, biases, and beliefs can stiffen our muscles in ways that make us uncomfortable in our body, absent ourselves from difficult emotions, and confuse our thinking. In short, we become fragmented, uncomfortable in our bodies, and unhappy in our being. The essence of any good yoga practice is to start the process of reintegration, so that breath, body, and mind start to feel more integrated.

Āsana and movement

We evolved to move, and the flesh and blood part of our being needs regular movement to maintain its functioning integrity, so it makes sense to use movement as the means to explore our sensory and perceptual world. This means a reasonable amount of consideration needs to be made about the kind of movements and *āsana*s you want to engage with. We clearly do not want to cause harm to ourselves, so movements that are congruent with our human morphology make sense, as well as those movements that will help us maintain an active life. These might include movements of the spine in flexion, side-bending, turning, and to some extent extension. It might also include the action of getting up off and down onto the floor, sitting in varied ways on the floor, and balancing. These should form the bedrock of our practice, and each teacher will devise ways of exploring such movements until they become familiar and comfortable to practise. I would add one more cate-gory to practice: movements that explicitly explore the relationship between support and muscle tension. These would include well-known *āsana*s like downward-facing dog, head balance base, and plank, which on their own have no functional relevance but when practised with sensitivity help illuminate the role our skeleton plays in supporting our body weight, thus relieving our muscles of much of the work of holding us up.

I stated earlier that the exercise or performance value of these practices is of secondary importance. I am interested, instead, in asking the following questions:

1. Am I clear about the intention of any movement?
2. Am I clearly doing what I intended to do? Am I adding anything?
3. Can I distinguish proprioception from nociception?
4. Can I distinguish between effort, tension, and relaxation?
5. Can I notice when I become uncomfortable, reflect on what happened when my state changed, and explore other ways of carrying out my intention with less discomfort?

Initially, all these things are framed within the context of a movement practice, but the same quality of focus can be applied to everyday life. Questions we might ask include:

1. Can I become clearer about what I am trying to achieve in any given situation?
2. Am I then doing that thing? Am I bringing more to it than I need to?
3. Do I notice when I go about my life whether it makes me unhappy?
4. Do I work enough, do I rest enough, and do I sometimes do too much when it is not necessary?
5. When I interact with the people and the world, can I get better at noticing when that interaction makes me feel uncomfortable? What happened at that point and how did I respond?

In all these cases, it is a feeling of either physical or mental discomfort that alerts us to the fact that something has happened that threatens our state of equilibrium or well-being. Simply getting better at asking these questions of yourself as you practice on the mat and go through life will help with adapting to ever-changing situations – which is, after all, what we are all faced with. A concrete example might be the way we approach plank pose. We start on all fours and then straighten out our legs behind us. During that process, many things can be noticed (or not, of course). When you straighten your legs, your support changes from largely bone to muscle and there is an increase in the effort to prevent the pelvis from collapsing to the floor. When transitions like this take place, it is often the time when we bring our habits to the movement, so it is helpful to straighten the legs very slowly so you can feel the gradual increase in muscular effort as your knees leave the floor. I think of this as the dimmer switch way of engaging muscles – a smooth, graded increase, and stopping when the appropriate amount of effort has been reached. If you straighten your legs quickly, the muscles turn on like a light switch. All the muscles come on at once, with no time to grade your effort and very likely adding habits such as holding the breath, or tightening the jaw. You can also pay close attention to what happens to the pelvis when you change your means of support, asking whether it moves up or down. Does it tilt anteriorly or even posteriorly? You want to be able to feel what is happening as you move from bony support to muscular support. You do not want a teacher to correct you after the act, as this takes away any potential for learning how to feel. If you notice something has changed unintentionally, the next time you do it try to notice when you bring the unintentional aspect of the movement in. That way, you slowly get to change your map of the movement.

If yoga becomes reduced to a version of exercise or performance a great deal can be missed. We may become stronger or be able to accomplish certain physical tasks, which will lift our spirits or enhance our self-esteem. These are both valuable things, but they ask no questions about why we feel the way we do, or how we get into difficulties physically, psychologically, or emotionally. Yoga can help us with this. We can become practised at noticing changes in our feeling state. We can get better at more finely granulating the sensations we perceive and therefore respond in a more nuanced way. We can get better at noticing when we cross the line between feeling well and unwell and what happened to initiate that change. It is a skill that when practised well has the power to change the course of your life. We respond more appropriately to the situations that arise in life and over time, we reduce the friction that may have existed, and we find more ease in ourselves and the world we inhabit.

8 —

HEAD, HEART, AND HANDS

Beverley Nolan

Beverley Nolan has been a yoga practitioner and teacher for more than 35 years. Like many of the teachers in this book (including Peter Blackaby), she began in the Iyengar tradition, but for the last 20 years she has been integrating somatic modalities such as IBMT (Integrative Bodywork and Movement Therapy), BodyMind Centering®, and the Feldenkrais® approach to intelligent movement into her practice and teaching.

She is the founder and director of studies at Barefoot Body Training, offering a somatic approach that is trauma-inclusive and open to exploring and understanding difference and accessibility. Her personal style combines a clear attention to experiential detail with intuitive and insightful questions.

For this piece, we asked her for a more personal reflection on the process of learning and integrating scientific knowledge into our lived experience of being a body. This piece invites you to witness the intimate process of incremental learning, humility, and self-reflection. It is a deep and at times vulnerable meditation on the role of the teacher in facilitating learning about anatomy through experience, while at the same time challenging hierarchies and supporting the discovery of each student's unique inner teacher.

As a teacher of long standing, I can vouch also for being a life-long learner. My desire for knowledge stems either from a growth mindset or a scarcity mindset. The former manifests as the impulse to follow my interests, deepening my existing knowledge. It results in a non-resistant learning encounter where I am in active participation with the teacher or facilitator and their material. The latter is more of an external impulse, manifesting either as the feeling that I don't know enough to maintain professional currency or as a requirement of ongoing education imposed by an accrediting organization. This results in a more resistant learning experience where I am typically less present and available to the offerings of the teacher.

My widest field of study has been anatomy, the development of human movement from foetus to child, and embryology. I am not an expert or academic researcher in any of these fields. My studies have evolved backwards, starting from a textbook separation of the body systems, through detailed experiential integration, arriving most recently at the sense of vibration in the chromosonal dance of conception and wondering how this might continue to resonate in my now adult body.

My decades of learning experiences have been both outside/in (head) and inside/out (heart), and I appreciate how the two approaches co-exist and affirm each other, neither ultimately assuming dominion over the other. As if to illustrate this, I recollect that during the earliest stages of my embryological growth, my heart was situated superior to my brain and through a process of relocation descended in front of my formless face to be held by my lungs and the accompanying breath. Both my heart and my head have been on top of things and below things, they know both as shared experiences in relation to one another. I also recall how the foetal development of my arms and hands have spiralled inwards to locate in front of my heart and how my foetal spine, cranium, and face, including what will be my organ of speech, all orient to my heart.

I choose to deconstruct three things now which I will classify in an embodied way and find that at the same time relate to the yogic paths described in the *Bhagavad Gītā*: head (thinking, *jñāna yoga*), heart (feeling, *bhakti yoga*) and hands/voice (doing, *karma yoga*). In terms of 'head' I reflect on knowledge as information that I acquire, process, and assimilate; for 'heart' I reflect on the first-hand felt-experience of knowledge that is lived through contemplative practice; for 'hands/voice' I reflect on the sharing of knowledge with others through teaching and facilitation.

THE DIALOGUE OF HEAD AND HEART

In my study and practice space at home, there are three shelves of anatomy books earmarked with sticky notes of all colours as well as two shelves of ring binders full of various course notes and a pile of art journals all arising from 20 years of somatic movement practices. I have long lists of research papers, links to YouTube animations and demonstrations, and a collection of Spotify playlists inspired by experiential anatomy. The windowsill in my study is currently home to anatomical models of the lower and upper limbs, a multicoloured skull model that I take apart from time to time with unvarying apprehension for its reconstruction, and a Huberman sphere. There is a basket of props in the corner, filled with resistance bands, soft balls (one half-filled with air, the other half-filled with water), bean bags, small weights, and a couple of rolled up face flannels. This disparate collection of objects and library of information offer me theoretical and practical pointers to understanding my own anatomy and physiology, but not as a subjective experience. This is the role of experiential study and play. Here my intellectual knowing evolves into a process of personal 'embodiment', a process of questions and affirmations, familiar and unfamiliar aspects of myself, memories, archetypes and images, and a rich and far-ranging landscape for the making of meaning.

Experiential anatomy (sometimes referred to as embodied anatomy) is the practice of bringing conscious awareness to body systems, structures, tissues, fluids, cells, and processes. It brings information offered up through text, images, models, and so on into first-hand exploration and experiences. I may get to know my skeletal system by handling anatomical models, studying diagrams, and observing animations of joint actions or the dynamic communication of osteoblasts[i] and osteoclasts.[ii] I may learn that bones are both light and strong, that they carry a history of my health and lifestyle that will exist beyond my lived days, that they are the containers of stem-cell-producing marrow, and that the alive bone in my body bears no resemblance in colour or substance to plastic models or samples found by forensic archaeologists – my living bone is rendered pink, fulsome and wet with inherent vitality.

All this I can 'learn', but in a way this learning is all in my head, in the hierarchical knowing of my nervous system, and while I gratefully receive this knowledge, it doesn't come alive, doesn't become personal, doesn't become relevant to the immediacy of my own body until I examine the relationship of this knowledge with the truth of my lived experience. Do I really experience my bones as being both light and strong? Is it possible to attune to and appreciate the dynamic nature of bone formation and absorption? What changes in my experience when I attend to the fertile nature

---

i   **osteoblast** [ŏs ′tē-ə-blăst′] A specialized bone cell that produces and deposits the matrix that is needed for the development of new bone and consists primarily of collagen fibres (www.dictionary. com/browse/osteoblast).

ii   **osteoclast** [ŏs ′tē-ə-klăst′] A specialized bone cell that absorbs bone, allowing for the deposition of new bone and maintenance of bone strength (www.dictionary.com/browse/osteoclast).

of the deep marrow? And, how is it to know that my bones carry a secret journal of my life: how I may be racially and sexually identified, where my ancestry is derived, the geographical and climactic setting of my lived life, the way I move, nourish myself, or experience disease and physical trauma? Indeed, if ever my bones are unearthed, they will even have recorded the number of my days.

What my skeletal remains won't say is how I perceive my bones as an embodiment of a mineral reality within the ocean of fluid that makes up the large part of my body, and how I understand this body that I have grown (from my embryological beginnings) as an expressive embodiment of the very Earth itself. My bone is the tissue that most directly knows what it is like to be a gravity-bound human. How I manage pathways of weight through my bones and attend to the nuanced dialogues occurring in my joint spaces invites my bones to find their way into right relationship with each other and with the external environment and, in this way, I may find the beauty (and the *sthira-sukha*, drawing on Patañjali[1]) of 'alignment' that no external voice can direct with unsubtle suggestions about shaping angles and stacking body parts. As Linda Hartley tells us:

> Connecting to the bones of our being connects us to that which is enduring, essential, ancient, grounding, and healing of soul and spirit. They connect us to life in its most fundamental, secure and lasting form. When we feel lost, ungrounded, insecure, cut loose without an anchor, the bones can help bring us home.[2]

Experiential enquiry reveals to me that each body system, structure, fluid, and process has the potential to express different aspects of myself. When I consciously inhabit my bony system, I experience one way of being that is not the same as when I consciously inhabit my blood system, my muscles, or my cellular membranes. Each gives rise to different qualities of movement or posture, to vocalizing in different ways, and to diverse seams of my unconscious that I can mine for associated language, images, stories, and ideas. Enquiry also makes space for knowing the 'mind' of my anatomical layers and features and as I get to know my body in these ways, I may access the possibility of integrating these aspects more knowingly into my conscious awareness. There exists the potential here to ameliorate my ability to respond to changing events, encounters, and environments. Do I want to meet you in the mind of my bones, or the mind of my blood, muscles, or membranes? How might you be meeting me? What would change in the way we speak, listen, or move together when we identify the anatomical ground of our shared presence? Returning to the wisdom of Linda Hartley, we find the following:

> Just as each body system expresses itself through a different quality and rhythm of movement, so too does each evoke a particular 'mind', a unique and recognisable energy or quality of awareness, perception and being that is expressed through the individual's presence and activity.[3]

A PHILOSOPHY OF THE BODY

The situating of the subject as the knower *and* the knowing is at the heart of experiential anatomy, and this resonates with my limited understanding of phenomenological thought. Phenomenology is the study of experience from the perspective of the experiencer – so far, so good! Experience includes sensory information as well as thought, imagination, memory, and emotion – again, good! Phenomenology came more clearly into form and gathered momentum at the beginning of the twentieth century, perhaps as a push-back against the dominance of Cartesian deductive reasoning (sovereignty of head over heart: *cogito ergo sum* – I think, therefore I am) which posited the duality of the body and mind to such an extent that one could exist without the other. It also gave primacy and status to scientific thought even though it was (is) unable to solve the most pressing of questions: 'the hard problem of consciousness' or the context in which thought is experienced: 'There is nothing that we know more intimately than conscious experience, but there is nothing that is harder to explain. All sorts of mental phenomena have yielded to scientific investigation in recent years, but consciousness has stubbornly resisted.'[4]

Phenomenologists can trace the evolutions of their varied thinking back to the writings of Edmund Husserl, and include in their ranks Martin Heidegger, who notably took issue with Descartes' focus on the *cogito* at the expense of unpacking the *sum*, and Maurice Merleau-Ponty, who in particular challenged the concept of the body as object, proposing that the body is necessary for all experiences and therefore its eternal presence renders it more subject than object:

> Visible and mobile, my body is a thing among things; it is caught in the fabric of the world, and its cohesion is that of a thing. But because it moves itself, sees, holds things in a circle around itself, things are an annex or prolongation of itself; they are encrusted into its flesh, they are part of its full definition; the world is made of the same stuff as the body.[5]

How can I bring my own felt-sense of the primacy and nonduality of the body-mind with my armchair understanding of phenomenological ideas to my study and my practice and my yoga? (And indeed, to an artful pedagogy for sharing yoga with others – see below.) If I reach for one of my preferred renderings of the *Yoga Sūtra of Patañjali*, a central text to most yoga teacher trainings, I find in the first breath of the writing an invocation to be ready and attentive to a presentation of the teachings of yoga, and then in the next breath I find the definition of what is meant here by the term 'yoga':[6] *yogaś citta-vṛtti-nirodhaḥ*.[7]

With the help of commentary texts, I can understand this statement as something contrary to my experiences of modern postural yoga (MPY)[8] where the focus of practice is typically dominated by organizing the body into a panoply of shapes (*āsana*s) and shape-sequences (*vinyāsa-krama*s). Patañjali is emphatic and transparent from the outset that the practice, psychology, and philosophy of yoga (based on the principles of Sāṃkhya[9] philosophy) is in fact about the uncoupling of the manifestations of *prakṛti* (matter/mind/body) from *puruṣa* (pure consciousness/soul). His implication is that the intellect, ego, and cognitive functions and capacity are not the home of consciousness, rather consciousness is a boundless context wherein all movements of the bodymind exist as impermanent experience. I can reach for an anatomical metaphor to ground these ideas in the shifting cellular currents in the vastness of my interstitium, a system that has no beginning or end, through which processes and communication signals come and go.

Patañjali also makes it clear that the preferred and most reliable way to confirm or contest the central tenet of yoga philosophy and arrive at right- or valid-knowledge (*pramāṇa*) is through direct experience (*pratyakṣa*), or experiential practice, if you will.[10] And while it would seem the body and the mind are extraneous to the purity of consciousness, it is as a bodymind that the practitioner will find their way into right-knowledge. In the introduction to Edwin Bryant's translation of the *Yoga Sūtras*, we find the following explanation:

> The origins of Yoga are rooted in direct perception of its subject matter, says the commentator Hariharananda Aranya. He too notes that Yoga is based not on the mere logical reasoning of the intellect but on direct experience, and in this regard differs from some of the other schools of orthodox thought, which are highly philosophical. Patañjali's Yoga Sūtras is more a psychosomatic technique than a treatise on metaphysics; the truth of Yoga cannot be experienced by inferential reasoning but only by direct perception.[11]

As Patañjali's text unfolds, I learn that there are a number of ways to cultivate the stillness of the mind and to arrive somewhere that is without suffering (essentially, the constructed sense of self that I call me/I is also a movement of the bodymind, and if the movement of the bodymind stills, ergo the me/I is no longer apparent and there can be no apparent experience of suffering). But, where is my mind? Can I locate it in the way that I can locate the presence of my bones? Can I witness my mind? Observe, sense, feel those turnings described in the second *sūtra* of the text? Is there anything from my experiential anatomy practices that could support this enquiry? Have I not indirectly been honing the skills of *pratyāhāra*, *dhāraṇā*, and *dhyāna* as described by Patañjali?[12]

Certainly, the fruits of my anatomy enquiries have been aided by my experience of the practice and the discipline of Authentic Movement, in which various modes of inner 'witnessing' are filtered and cultivated.[13] I might track where I am in space, how I am moving or not moving, how I have arranged my body as a result of attending to physical sensations. I might also track emotional content that arises in my moving, or open my awareness to my imagination and notice image, archetype, story, or myth arising. I might also be open to the idea or experience of the collective field or the transpersonal.

As an example, when I experience something that I describe as pain, in my conscious witnessing of this set of sensations certain choices arise. That is to say, as a consequence of my inner witness demerging from the immediacy of the experience, pathways of agency appear. I might stop whatever I think is causing the pain, I might modulate what I am doing to reduce the intensity, I might choose to savour the sensation as an affirmation of being alive, or of bringing me back from a place of dissociation, and I might also notice that my inner witness does not itself experience the pain but is perhaps offering up the closest personal experience of clear being-ness that my personal bodymind can know: 'The process of embodiment is a being process, not a doing process, not a thinking process.'[14]

HANDS AND VOICE: TEACHING AND FACILITATION

My personal integration of head and heart learning through experiential enquiries (hands) has led to an ongoing process of meaning-making, as well as a deepening of my own contemporary yogic enquiry into the unknowable nature of being. In some ways this is more than enough, in other ways the impulse to continue sharing in the world of somatic education remains. However, I experience a tension in myself between the power dynamic and intrinsic conditions of instructional learning spaces for yoga (head and hands) where individuals respond to clear cues and timings, and those of a participative pedagogy (head, heart, and hands) where individuals have the opportunity to be more self-directed in their embodied learning process. Alongside this professional tension, I am acutely aware of the reality of my situation as a white, middle-class, neurotypical, cis-woman. As such, how am I limited (or am I limiting) in the ways that I might share knowledge and make experiential enquiry accessible to bodyminds that may not look like mine, express like mine, or have lived a life like mine? What are the ways I might contribute meaningfully to the equitable dissemination of experiential practices? These are the questions I live, and this is the place to start the enquiry from. Rilke's advice to 'a young poet' is apt to remember here:

> I would like to beg you dear Sir, as well as I can, to have patience with everything unresolved in your heart and to try to love the questions them-selves as if they were locked rooms or books written in a very foreign lan-guage. Don't search for the answers, which could not be given to you now, because you would not be able to live. And the point is to live everything. Live the questions now. Perhaps then, someday far in the future, you will gradually, without even noticing it, live your way into the answer.[15]

Certainly, I do find myself sharing anatomy information (head) so that someone might helpfully learn more about their body. I teach techniques (head) so that someone might better functionally organize and move their body in and out of agreed shapes and sequences. I can also stratify content (head) into beginners (knows nothing or little), intermediate (knows more), and advanced (knows even more), and some teachers (not so much me) will correct and adjust towards an aesthetic or required representation of a shape (head). These are the characteristics of a teacher as a mediator of knowledge and skills using head methodologies. I notice this in myself when I spend most of my time at the front of the room, stick to my lesson plan come what may, and refer to my content as a class and the people attending as students. I also find I am more in this mode when I am teaching online or pre-recording a class, and why I have struggled with these formats. With head-based pedagogy, there is a sense that the body, breath, and mind are to be controlled by the voice of a teacher.

When I teach using heart methodologies, I begin to engage the people in the room in their direct experience by offering contrasting experiences that they might evaluate for themselves. 'Try placing your feet this way and notice how it affects the position of your pelvis and your experience of comfort or discomfort. Now try placing your feet this way and check in again...do you have a preference?' In asking them to notice their own experience I might also point out how it might be different from mine or that of their neighbours, and I will sincerely mean it and be unafraid of being without an answer when I ask if anyone has a question. I may still call this a class and the people there the students but there is time and space for their voices and their unique experiences. I find I am likely to move around the room and among the students, and not to see my lesson plan through to the letter, and there is a permission from myself to free-style my content in response to what happens in the space. In this move towards a more participative pedagogy (possibly andragogy would be more appropriate), there is a sense that the body, breath, and mind are being guided by the outer teacher and that there is active encouragement for the inner teacher to find their voice.

Blending together head, heart, and hands methodologies has the potential to create an even more integrative and participative learning experience for all concerned. It begins to shift the yoga teacher's role to include the facilitation of multiple unique experiences as well as the sharing of relevant knowledge and opportunities for the practice of skills. It's true to say that a hierarchical dynamic remains, as the teacher-facilitator continues to hold the boundaries of time, overall content, and safety. But facilitation shifts the balance towards a contextual responsiveness from the participants, so that each class, which might be renamed session or circle or gathering, evolves organically. In this approach, my lesson plan becomes a series of seeds for enquiry based around some contractual agreements made with the consensus of the group. This might, for example, allow for individuals to find their own practice space in the room, to use or not use a mat, to make intuitive sounds, or to follow their own inner movement impulses. It will always include time for sharing together at the beginning and end of the session. For myself, I am likely to hold an anchor of constancy by positioning myself in one space in the room, and to be witnessing my own experiences in response to the participants almost as much as I witness them. I will cast seeds of enquiry into the collective space and await the alchemy of the people, the place, and the moment.

Yoga class teaching in the manner of facilitation aligns with my understanding of that which is being pointed to by Patañjali: it is not something that is taught by another, rather something that is pointed to by another, since what is being pointed to cannot be 'known' in the ordinary sense of the word. In certain respects, facilitation acknowledges that all the science in the world, all the teachers in the world, all the philosophers in the world can never know the first-hand experience of another bodymind, yet each offers signposts and pathways to the recognition of this. Facilitating a space for a shared yoga potentially allows for the movement from, to, and between learning and experiencing so that each of those who are present might get the chance to glimpse, or taste, or sniff the unlearnable, the unknowable.

TEACHING, AGENCY, AND TRAUMA

9 —

TRAUMA, YOGA, AND SPIRITUAL ABUSE

Amelia Wood

Amelia Wood is a doctoral candidate at SOAS, University of London, researching spiritual abuse in modern transnational yoga communities. Her research aims to centre survivor voices and resist epistemic injustice. She completed her MA in the traditions of yoga and meditation at SOAS in 2015, specializing in representations of women in pre-modern yoga practices.

Amelia has been teaching yoga and working in the yoga industry since 2010. Her teaching focuses on the therapeutic application of yoga to the individual, breath awareness, and mindful, meditative movements. She now trains yoga teachers, drawing from her own teaching and academic experience and expertise.

For this piece, once again, we asked for more than a simple introduction to what trauma is and how it manifests in a yoga practice. Rather than confining herself to the rather speculative science around bodies and trauma, instead Amelia offers us a history of 'trauma-informed care' as a theme of yoga practice and culture. This chapter problematizes the diagnostics and politics of trauma-informed approaches, whilst affirming the place of trauma survivors in general yoga classes. This blurred edge between recreational, and spiritual, and therapeutic forms of yoga practice is equally applicable to other kinds of accessibility – our classes should be as accessible as we can make them, if only because a wide diversity of students, with and without diagnoses, will find their way to our classes.

This chapter also examines the structural nature of trauma: how access to healing spaces is limited by marginalization of various forms, and how marginalized groups are often the most subject to traumatic experiences. Most importantly, Amelia also reminds us of the trauma and abuse that occur within yoga spaces, and gifts us the academic term 'spiritual abuse' to recognize the entangled impact of multiple forms of abuse in one. Abuse in yoga settings is always more than financial abuse, sexual abuse, or physical abuse. It is always complicated by the meaning and fulfilment students also find in those spaces.

For obvious reasons, this section comes with a strong content note for mentions of abuse and suicide.

When I began teaching yoga and working as a yoga therapist over a decade ago the phrase 'trauma-informed' did not come up. When talking to my supervisor it was understood some clients had been 'traumatized', but it was never suggested that, in response, I should take a specifically trauma-informed approach: it was not at the forefront of our lexicon. When this dawned on me recently, I found it so unbelievable that I had to double-check with someone from my cohort – had I misremembered my entire training experience?[i]

Trauma-informed training courses for yoga teachers, both online and in person, in the English-speaking yoga world are now plentiful: why has this changed? The opening to Judith Herman's seminal book *Trauma and Recovery* (1992) offers some insight. She writes, 'The study of psychological trauma has a curious history – one of episodic amnesia.'[1] In the past, headway has been made, an abundant tradition created, and then, 'it has been periodically forgotten and must be periodically reclaimed'.[2] We are currently in a period of reclaiming – the trauma-informed discourse has resurfaced significantly enough for it to have an impact on the yoga industry. But who gets to reclaim and utilize trauma-informed methods and practices? From whom and for whom are they being reclaimed? How do some trauma-informed modalities participate in reinforcing power structures and how can we, as yoga teachers, reduce the possibility of replicating harm? In this chapter I will briefly talk about the history of trauma-informed care, and address questions of power and ownership, and what relationship such things have to the business of teaching yoga.

---

i   Thanks to Zoe Martin for being my sounding board.

A BRIEF HISTORY OF TRAUMA-INFORMED CARE

After the First and Second World Wars, soldiers with unexplained physical or emotional disorders were deemed 'shell shocked': a term that appeared in *The Lancet*, a British medical journal, in 1915.[3] Such inexplicable symptoms included fatigue, insomnia, nightmares, palpitations, joint and muscle pain, loss of voice or hearing. Doctors struggled to adequately diagnose and military authorities struggled to accept such a reaction in their soldiers.[4] Many believed they should not be treated as patients but 'court-martialled' or 'dishonourably discharged'.[5] They were, as Herman aptly summarizes, acting like women who, in the past, would have been categorized as 'hysterical'.[6]

In the late nineteenth century, decades before the term 'shell shock' was coined, 'hysteria' in women was studied seriously for the first time by the French neurologist Jean-Martin Charcot.[7] Charcot documented symptoms carefully, systematically, and exhaustively. By the 1880s, he – reasonably – concluded that such 'symptoms were psychological'.[8]

Pierre Janet and Sigmund Freud, two of Charcot's followers, sought to surpass his work – in the 1880s, this process involved both doctors listening to women with what Herman calls a 'devotion and respect unparalleled before or since'.[9] Unsurprisingly, this resulted in fruitful discoveries – Janet and Freud independently concluded that hysteria was caused by psychological trauma. Freud continued his investigations into the sexual lives of women. What he heard, repeatedly, were frequent accounts of sexual assault, abuse, and incest. Troubled by his findings, Freud was reluctant to admit that abusive acts perpetrated against children were as prevalent as his own research suggested. In the 1890s he stopped listening to women and 'out of the ruins of the traumatic theory or hysteria' he 'created psychoanalysis'. Herman notes that 'the dominant psychological theory of the next century was founded in the denial of women's reality' and sexual exploitation was re-imagined, by Freud, as fantasy.[10]

It was only during and in the aftermath of trench warfare that society remembered and reclaimed the concept of psychological trauma. Following shell shock, the term post-traumatic stress disorder (PTSD) was coined in response to soldiers returning from the Vietnam War (1955–1975). In 1980 the American Psychiatric Association included the term in their diagnostic manual and, once formally recognized, studies regarding the prevalence of PTSD could be conducted.[11] The term PTSD is, however, still contested in medical circles. 'Disorder' suggests a maladaptive response in those exposed to trauma. But are distress, anxiety, hyper-alertness, rather than being abnormal, relatively normal reactions to abnormal situations?[12] Conversely, without a term as a means to diagnose, the medical community cannot study patients, nor offer treatments.

We know now that the experience of trauma and possible subsequent PTSD is not limited to war veterans but that – in the words of Bessel van der Kolk – it can happen 'to us, our friends, our families, and our neighbours'.[13] Part of Kolk's work as a medical doctor has been to create a consensus regarding the diagnosis of developmental trauma disorder, to capture the reality of the clinical presentations of children and adolescents exposed to chronic interpersonal trauma in order to utilize effective interventions. People who have experienced ongoing danger and maltreatment as children are currently under-served by the current diagnostic system. In 2009 a consensus of criteria to diagnose developmental trauma disorder was proposed by the National Child Traumatic Stress Network taskforce. Their work intends to describe the clinically significant symptoms exhibited following complex trauma in children and adolescents. Such symptoms do not only include PTSD but also physiological dysregulation, attention and behaviour dysregulation, and functional impairment.[14]

YOGA, TRAUMA, AND TRAUMA-INFORMED CARE

Bessel van der Kolk's work (amongst others) indicates that the study of trauma and trauma-informed care is not only being remembered and reclaimed but that it has reached a point where it is in conversation with, and being integrated by, other disciplines and industries, including yoga.

When offering group classes in any setting people who have experienced complex traumas will invariably attend our classes. They may not disclose the fact of their trauma to you, as the teacher. They may not be at your class to address their trauma. They may not be on a journey of healing, or have a diagnosis.

Given that trauma-informed care has had a patchy history, it is unsurprising that individuals are still often misdiagnosed. They may have been brushed off as a child with behavioural difficulties, or simply not been believed: a lack of appropriate diagnosis does not deny the experience of trauma. Thus, whilst the role of the yoga teacher is not to diagnose, we must be aware that trauma is a common experience and that people who have had traumatic experiences will attend our classes.

In my early work as a yoga teacher and therapist, I was certain that my offerings could be categorized in two distinct ways – the recreational and the therapeutic. General group classes in gyms and yoga studios were recreational.

I assumed attendees were there to enjoy an experience rather than to address a particular issue. Classes offered a connection between the body and mind, a moment of mindfulness and relaxation, something vaguely spiritual but not religious. If an attendee had a specific need I adapted poses to accommodate, as I had been taught to do. In contrast, group classes for specialist conditions and one-to-one yoga therapy sessions were more actively therapeutic. They were spaces in which people acknowledged specific and individual needs that I, as their yoga therapist, could address.

As I got to know those participating in the (recreational) group classes my categorization system collapsed. I learnt that recreational and therapeutic can coexist and that it is not for me to assume why someone is attending a class. I found that many had experienced trauma – lost family members, suffered serious illness, been diagnosed and medicated for mental health conditions, or experienced other traumas I would never be party to.[i] Many could not, or did not want to, come to me on a one-to-one basis as a yoga therapy client. I believe this was mostly for structural reasons – lack of funds, an absence of support, and continual marginalization.

Structural prejudice exists within the medical establishment and in wider society. To receive clinical treatment, one must be diagnosed. In order to receive a correct diagnosis, however, such a diagnosis must first exist. We can see from Kolk's *The Body Keeps The Score*, from Jones and Wessely's work on military psychiatry, and Freud's response to his patients, that symptoms can, and have historically, been misinterpreted. Reaching a consensus on conditions, diagnostic methods, and clinical treatments is a lengthy and often contentious process. Furthermore, in order to gain any knowledge on suffering and trauma the medical establishment is reliant on those who have survived traumatic experiences. A significant amount of knowledge comes from survivors themselves. We have seen from Freud's work that even when survivors are listened to and understood, the medical authority can claim a survivor's truth is fantasy.

In addition to the power imbalance within medical institutions, external power imbalances are at play. Herman writes that when 'the victim is already devalued (a woman, a child)' it is likely that she will 'find that the most traumatic events of her life take place outside the realm of socially validated reality. Her experience becomes unspeakable'.[15] For whom are such things unspeakable and who benefits from this silence around trauma caused by violence? Society privileges those who are able-bodied, white, cisgender,

---

i   These descriptions are generalizations and do not represent any specific individuals.

heteronormative, male presenting, and who have relative wealth. Those who experience trauma are often already structurally marginalized – they live in vulnerable situations that those with more power can exploit. Once traumatized, one is further marginalized. And if, prior to experiencing trauma, the individual is not in a position of relative marginalization it is likely they will then experience marginalization: this is a circular problem. They cannot, therefore, necessarily access a clinical diagnosis or treatment with the medical institution.

There are a number of ways that we can address this circular problem. There are an ever-increasing number of trauma-informed courses out there for yoga teachers. You could enrol onto a training, align yourself with specialists who have developed theories by studying survivors, follow their protocol, and proclaim you are trauma-informed. You might add new classes to your schedule and advertise them as being a 'safe space'. But remember: people who have experienced trauma are already attending your classes. Teach who is in front of you. Teach and accommodate those who have experienced trauma as you would someone who has a back problem but know that, whilst the latter might casually inform you of their condition, a traumatized individual might not be able to name, or claim, their own experiences. Your group class might be the only opportunity some people have to therapeutically connect with their whole self. Marginalization and lack of privilege are social constructs. As a small act of resistance, we can reframe all our classes to accommodate people who have experienced trauma due to marginalization, or are marginalized due to trauma, in an attempt to disrupt the circle.

TRAUMA WITHIN THE YOGA INDUSTRY

There is another reason why we, as yoga teachers, must be trauma-aware: people have and will continue to experience trauma, abuse, and violence within yoga contexts. Yoga is not exceptional or immune from causing participants trauma, because yoga classes and communities exist within and not outside the fabric of society.

As it stands, one would be hard pressed to find a modern, transnational yoga lineage that has not been party to allegations of abuse. In addition, it is often impossible to extract reported instances of emotional and psychological from sexual abuse, or financial abuse from physical abuse – they are entangled and enable one another to occur. As such, in my own research, I use the umbrella term: spiritual abuse.[16]

All of the following examples occurred from the late twentieth century onwards. Some came to light before, and some after, the popularization of #metoo in October 2017, after its inception by Tarana Burke several years prior. All occurred within organizations that were, and in some cases still are, popular and prevalent in the English-speaking yoga world and beyond – Bikram Yoga, Anusara Yoga, Satyananda Yoga, Ashtanga and Sivananda Yoga. It is important to acknowledge that abuse from within yoga communities is not far removed, or separate from, our experience as yoga teachers but part of our wider industry.

Abuse was perpetrated within the Satyananda Yoga community in the 1970s and 80s, but it was in the context of the Australian Royal Commission into Institutional Responses to Child Sexual Abuse that details were brought to light.[17] In 2012 Julia Gillard, the former Australian prime minister, instigated the Royal Commission and it ran from 2013 to 2017. The commission heard that sexual, financial, physical, and emotional abuse was perpetrated within the Satyananda Yoga ashram at Mangrove Mountain against children and adults. As part of the ritual initiation into the ashram, members had to give up familial ties and change their names, and were encouraged not to contact the outside world. Often, this resulted in children being separated from parents. The ashram took control of child welfare payments, and minors were left vulnerable. It was reported that Swami Akhandananda, the head of Mangrove Mountain, took advantage of this and sexually abused several children in his care. Jyoti, who gave testimony as part of the Royal Commission, reported that he threatened to kill her if she told anyone of his abusive acts. Despite this emotional manipulation she did, eventually, disclose the abuse to two adults within the Satyananda Yoga community, but they failed to act appropriately. As devotees, they believed so strongly that Akhandananda represented God they were unable to hear her truth. Jyoti was, as Herman would put it, devalued, or marginalized, for being a child. Financial abuse (the redirection of child welfare payments and lack of financial means for children to escape) enabled sexual and emotional abuse (as they had no one to protect them from the Swami, a predator), which was supported by hierarchical power structures.

More recently, in 2012, John Friend, who founded Anusara Yoga in the US, was exposed on an anonymous website for abusing his position of power. The website released video footage of Friend incriminating himself of professional misconduct. It was claimed he committed financial abuse and misled several women with whom he engaged in sexual relationships. Shortly after, in 2013, Bikram Choudhury, the founder of Bikram Yoga, was also accused of abuse.[18] Three former students and one former employee filed lawsuits against

Choudhury and his yoga school in the US. The cases included accusations of sexual assault, sexual abuse, battery, psychological abuse, withholding of wages, and a culture of silencing and manipulation.

Since the popularization of #metoo, countless individuals have come forward about abuse they've experienced in yoga contexts. Rachel Brathen, known on social media as 'Yoga Girl', collected hundreds of these stories and posted them on her website in 2019.[19] Matthew Remski's 2019 book – *Practice and All Is Coming: Abuse, Cult Dynamics, and Healing in Yoga and Beyond* – details survivor accounts of alleged abuse carried out by Patthabi Jois, the founder of the Ashtanga Yoga organization.[20] Allegations suggest that Jois did this in plain sight, throughout his career, in the late twentieth century. Several of those who came forward – most notably Karen Rain and Jubilee Cooke – had already spoken about the abuse they suffered, but received new attention in light of the online #metoo movement. In 2019, Julie Salter wrote a social media post that detailed the abuse she experienced in the Sivananda Yoga organization.

There have been very few consequences, in terms of justice for victims and survivors who have come forward, regarding the cases listed above. Mangrove Mountain offered an apology and compensation to those who gave testimonies as part of the Royal Commission, but the central Satyananda Yoga organization has issued no such apology or acknowledgement of harm. John Friend ceased to be the head of Anusara Yoga but continues to teach yoga online and in Denver, Colorado, as I write in 2022. The Sivananda Yoga ashrams continue to receive students and train hundreds of yoga teachers a year. In response to Julie Salter's revelations of abuse, more women came forward and Project SATYA (Sivananda – Accountability – Truth Seeking – Yogic Action; www.projectsatya.org) was co-founded by Angela Gollat and Jens Augspurger, to stand in solidarity with survivors. Investigations by Project SATYA found that the Sivananda organization covered up abuse and sexual misconduct. Mysore, India, continues to be the centre of Ashtanga Yoga, and it remains a popular class on yoga studio schedules. Some studios formerly associated with Bikram Yoga have closed or re-branded as hot yoga studios, but many still exist. Choudhury left the US for a few years, after judgement had been entered against him in a number of legal cases but before any compensation had been paid to the claimant, but he began training yoga teachers again in 2019, and on International Yoga Day in 2022 an online class led by Choudhury was advertised widely on social media.

The list I have presented is not exhaustive – there have been cases of abuse reported from former members of other yoga communities, such as Iyengar yoga and Jivamukti yoga; Philip Deslippe has written about the complex abuses of power within 3HO, commonly known as Kundalini yoga.[21] Given space limitations, here is not the place to continue listing details, but there is plenty of publicly available and creditable information available to those who wish to read more.

CONCLUSION

Given the prevalence of abuse both in society at large and from within our own industry it is vital that we, as yoga teachers, take seriously the notion that people who have experienced trauma already attend our classes. It is likely that some victims or survivors sought out yoga communities as a place and means to heal, only to be met with further violence and violations. It is therefore possible that people attending your yoga classes are in search of healing from trauma, experienced from both within and outside of yoga contexts.

To avoid repeating what Judith Herman calls the curious history and episodic amnesia of trauma and its associated care, we must engage with the concept of trauma awareness.

We must continually reclaim the idea that yoga teachers can offer a space for survivors in which they do not need to disclose traumatic incidents but can still engage in the process of healing. What can we do within yoga spaces not only to reduce the likelihood of re-traumatization, but to support healing? Is it possible to be trauma-aware in community settings and to reduce the replication of power imbalances even if, like me, you trained before the concept of trauma-informed yoga became popular in our industry?

10 —

PERSON-CENTRED TEACHING FOR TRAUMA

Harriet McAtee and Laura Wilson

Like earlier pieces in this book, this chapter has arisen out of significant collaboration. Theo and Harriet (along with Amelia, from the previous chapter) co-teach a course for yoga teachers called 'Yoga, Trauma & the Nervous System'. The recordings and transcripts of this course formed the basis for two blog posts that Harriet worked on with her long-term writing collaborator, Miranda Weindling.[1] But when we originally conceived of that course, we were hoping that Laura Wilson would also be able to join us.

Laura is the founding director of Edinburgh Community Yoga, a not-for-profit social enterprise with a focus on promoting accessible and inclusive yoga in underserved communities. She is also a minded yoga therapist specializing in trauma-informed yoga for mental health. She has been practising yoga since 2004 and teaching in mainstream settings as well as in collaboration with third-sector organizations, NHS services, and criminal justice services since 2011.

Laura is a survivor, practitioner, yoga teacher, and therapist, with a gift for understanding the complex relationship between the experiences we have, the subsequent patterning laid down in our nervous system and subconscious, and the interplay between body and mind in integrating these experiences. She is motivated by a deep faith in our ability to integrate, process, let go, and reframe, and finds the rich tapestry of practices offered in yoga to be an extraordinary set of tools for navigating life as a human being.

This chapter combines the above blog posts with significant

insights from Laura's long history of working in this field. In our experience, it is rare for trauma trainings to be led by professionals who are also survivors. We believe this gives us insights that are rarely included when survivors are only the subjects, rather than the co-creators of care.

This chapter centres on personal agency, and its role in making yoga teaching more sensitive to the experiences of trauma. It de-emphasizes simplistic ideas of 'healing' in favour of student-centred experiences of empowerment, and evaluates the existing culture of trauma-informed yoga trainings in the light of this shift in focus. The chapter ends with Harriet providing a set of enquiries for those interested in pursuing further training, and guidelines for the responsibilities, scope of practice, and interpersonal boundaries that help ensure any yoga teaching environment is truly trauma-informed.

Whilst this chapter does not contain references to specific incidents, a content note for the general themes of abuse and trauma still applies.

Putting trauma into words is no easy feat, but there is one idea that speaks to many elements of trauma, covering both how it is experienced and how we might understand it: trauma is complex. The lived experience of trauma is complex, the medical establishment's understanding of trauma is complex, the social and cultural contexts of trauma are complex, and the intersection of trauma and yoga is also complex. So, given this complex nature, how do we navigate trauma in the yoga space?

This chapter is divided into two parts. First, we'll be exploring how we can navigate trauma in our teaching through what we believe is the one essential key principle for providing a much safer space for trauma survivors: agency. We'll uncover why agency matters above all else and unpack how a yoga setting can help restore, emphasize, and create space for personal agency through the lenses of triggers, consent, and healing. Then we will offer practical advice on how to integrate our understanding of agency into our teaching.

Second, we'll be providing a framework in which to locate this understanding in the existing culture of trauma-informed yoga. We'll explore how trauma-informed teacher trainings need to improve for them to be safe, effective, and meaningful in supporting trauma survivors. We'll also consider our responsibility as yoga teachers when teaching trauma-informed classes.

Drawing upon our experience both as survivors and yoga teachers, we will break down some of the bigger theoretical concepts and discourse surrounding trauma-informed teaching into real-life practice. Taking the complex and nuanced theory of trauma and consent into a yoga space against the daunting and often volatile backdrop of power dynamics, social justice, and diversity and inclusion requires an enormous amount of bravery, skill, and consideration. But it is worth the effort. As we will discuss, it is important to make the distinction between spaces where we are explicitly inviting people who have active complex post-traumatic stress disorder (C-PTSD), and spaces where we can't assume the absence of people with active C-PTSD. For the first, it is essential that we have a substantial number of hours of training in the intricacies of trauma-informed practice. For the second, less formal training may be required, but all yoga teachers should know that traumatized people show up in all yoga spaces. People who are hurt, dysregulated, and overwhelmed are very often drawn to practices such as yoga. They are open to its transformational and healing potential. Importantly, however, they are also vulnerable to the potentially harmful and even re-traumatizing effects of the practice and the culture around it, if it is offered unskilfully. If you are a community-focused teacher who is actively seeking to teach groups who are unlikely to find their way into a yoga studio, many of the people you teach will be traumatized, marginalized, and pathologized in their distress. Agency and empowerment become even more imperative in those cases.

No one trains to be a yoga teacher to do harm. We all have the desire to do good, to share what we have found supportive of this extraordinary practice with others. However, holding that intention is not enough on its own. This chapter aims to support you as a yoga teacher to integrate and embody your learning into practical and supportive suggestions for quality, people-sensitive teaching.

WHAT IS AGENCY?

A sense of agency, or personal agency, is our ability to feel in control or be able to take action. A nice, although not entirely inclusive, definition of agency comes from psychologist and researcher Dr James Moore: 'When we make voluntary actions we tend not to feel as though they simply happen to us, instead we feel as though we are in charge. The sense of agency refers to this feeling of being in the driving seat when it comes to our actions.'[2] The key ideas here are 'voluntary actions' and the transition from something 'happen[ing] to us' to being 'in charge of our actions' in situations. Sometimes control is painted as a dirty word – and in some instances it is – but when it comes to trauma survivors, being able to restore a level of control over all or some aspects of a situation is paramount to feeling safe. Exerting control can help in reclaiming a part of one's self.

Agency is often experienced as a sliding scale: we may not always feel in complete control of a situation, but we might feel like we at least have a say in the situation. Alternatively, we may not be able to control absolutely everything in a situation, but we may be able to identify areas that we can control. A sense of personal agency is integral for everyone, in and beyond a yoga space. But the role of agency takes on particular significance for trauma survivors.

The relationship between trauma and agency

A traumatic experience represents a multi-faceted loss of agency. The traumatic event is a physically, emotionally, and/or psychologically threatening event. The individual's response to this event is some form of emotional overwhelm. The consequence of this – both whilst experiencing the trauma and in its aftermath – is a threatened or diminished sense of self coupled with some form of emotional dysregulation. Importantly, the individual's response to the traumatic situation was helpful and essential at that moment as it ensured their survival. When the traumatic experience becomes embedded, the pain, distress, and similar responses experienced as a consequence can be triggered and re-lived as flashbacks, physical sensations, intrusive thoughts, or nightmares. Traumatic responses and triggers are not fixed. How and what is experienced can change over time. Triggers and responses can have different intensities: they may be completely debilitating and overwhelming, or be manageable, albeit uncomfortable. As Amelia has written in the previous chapter, those who experience trauma are significantly more likely to belong to vulnerable or marginalized groups. The more disenfranchised you are by society, the more at risk you are for multiple traumatic events. This includes people of colour, the LGBTQI+ community, immigrants, women, and anyone who lives in a marginalized body.

All of this equates to a loss, threat to, or removal of agency. In many ways what survivors are tasked with doing for the rest of their lives is finding ways to restore and reconnect to their agency. The symptoms and manifestations of traumatic experiences present on a vast spectrum of physical affect, behaviours, and emotional responses. This ranges from survivors whose behaviours are so prevalent in society they have been normalized in our culture, to those who are highly pathologized, medicalized, and hospitalized by their presentations.

Given that our responses to trauma are unique, a checklist of potentially helpful things to introduce or remove will not ensure a trauma-informed yoga space. However, as all trauma survivors share a loss of agency, creating a yoga class where agency is emphasized can create pathways for students to heal in meaningful ways. In order to do this we do not need to re-invent yoga. Instead, we must consciously decide how to offer this practice in a way that leans into the tools already available, and consciously leans away from the approaches that move us further from accessing agency. Offering choice instead of commands, suggestion over direction, empowerment over control, and the collaborative over the performative gives students genuine permission to take care of themselves. Nonetheless, experiencing agency doesn't always feel comfortable. For many people, being able to freely say or do what they need, and their actions being respected, can feel odd or overwhelming or even terrifying.

TRAUMA AND TRIGGERS

Trauma-informed yoga trainings often focus on removing or minimizing potential triggers. Of course, no one wants to trigger a survivor. And yet, if survivors themselves can't control for or explain every trigger, how can you, external to the survivors' experience, be expected to do that for them? Triggers are complex, chaotic, and dynamic. Triggers can change over time. Triggers are very often unexpected. A survivor may go to extraordinary lengths to avoid triggers, but as any survivor will tell you, they are a fact of life.

In a trauma-informed yoga class, this means creating a space in which regaining agency is possible. If your yoga class is a space where students are actively encouraged and supported in practising their agency, then if they are triggered by something in class, they are in an environment where they can do what they need to support themselves. Trauma survivors are strong and resilient. You don't need to wrap them up in cotton wool or act overly apologetic for everything you are uncertain about. Instead, recognize your students' strength, resilience, and how much they know themselves. Chances are they have been living with their trauma for weeks, if not years or decades, and they have strategies for managing their triggers.

It is not the end of the world to trigger a survivor. What is unacceptable is to make a bad situation worse by trying to control or minimize their experience. What a trauma survivor does not need is to be triggered when they have been explicitly told they won't be. We cannot account for every aspect of the student experience, but we can establish a space where our students feel able, perhaps even empowered, to do whatever it is they need to do to take care of themselves.

Consent

In all situations, we should aim for consent to be informed, enthusiastic, and ongoing. Many survivors give away their agency as a survival strategy. For these students, although they may express consent, it may not always be genuinely empowered, enthusiastic, or freely given – so it is not consent.

We often think of consent as saying yes enthusiastically, but for survivors saying a happy, confident, guilt- or anxiety-free 'no' is arguably more powerful. The ability to comfortably change your mind and withdraw consent needs to be celebrated. All decisions in a yoga space should be informed and should be able to be met with a confident 'not today'. As soon as a student walks into your class they are saying yes to being there. This means they can also say yes to walking out again. We as teachers need to become comfortable with being rejected. We have to genuinely encourage a response of 'no thank you'. We may enjoy the feeling of people in the room looking for our attention, our touch, our reassurance, our time. And if this is the case, we must be conscious about how this dynamic affects the agency of our students.

Clearly it is important that we find ways for people to give informed consent moment to moment. But this is not a simple thing to get right, particularly if working with people who already feel small, marginalized, underrepresented, traumatized, and therefore unlikely to feel the capacity to speak up. Historically, 'trauma-informed' yoga spaces have often removed any possibility of teachers touching students. In many situations, this is still probably the wisest choice. But it is always important to consider how we go about offering touch in a way that will work for everyone. Hopefully, as we build a relationship with someone we teach, we will develop a greater ability to establish consent easily and fluidly, moment to moment.

One unbelievably helpful thing you can do to help your students make informed choices is make your class descriptions clear. Class descriptions should cover what to expect in the class, and identify who the class is appropriate for and what equipment is needed. A class description is essentially a contract in which you detail what is on offer, and potential students can consent, decline, or ask questions about any elements of the description.

Healing

The relationship between yoga and healing is complex and our thinking around how these concepts are related is often entangled in damaging ways. We believe that yoga may be a part of our healing journey, but healing is not the goal of yoga. We may heal through yoga, but yoga does not heal us. Yoga can help us uncover personal healing, but yoga and healing are not done to us.

The concepts of healing, therapies, and therapeutics are found more and more in yoga spaces. But yoga is not a drug or a tried-and-tested medical intervention. The studies that have been conducted on yoga are often rife with limitations. Although some studies on yoga are interesting, therapeutic medical trials shouldn't be our driving source of knowledge in the yoga community.

At the intersection of yoga, trauma, and healing, once again the most effective thing yoga can provide is a space where people can practise consent and agency. Exploring and practising yoga skills in a community setting that actively encourages you to express agency and consent can be profoundly healing. But in our opinion, the word 'healing' should be left out of descriptions of the trauma-informed yoga space entirely. Instead, a trauma-informed yoga setting should outline that it is a judgement-free space where trauma survivors are welcome, where different modalities relating to yoga will be explored, and where the individual will be respected and welcomed to choose what they do and don't want to do.

PRACTICAL WAYS TO ENCOURAGE AGENCY IN A YOGA CLASS

Pretty much all these elements are appropriate for any yoga class, whether specific to trauma survivors or not. These tips are also good practice in general for making your classes more inclusive.

- **Before the first session, provide clear and informative class descriptions.** If the class is in-person include images and even a video of the space.
- **Give choices and options.** The choice to rest or move. Options in the poses. Choices not to do a specific pose, meditation, or *prāṇāyāma* practice. The option to leave the room, no questions asked, for whatever reason. Too much choice can be confusing and overwhelming, so make it clear and simple.
- **Don't just say everything is a choice or optional.** Describe what that might look like or mean, and how taking rest and bathroom breaks, and leaving the room as needed is encouraged.
- **Use invitational language,** as opposed to instructions so your students are aware they are being invited to try something or turn it down, as opposed to being told what to do.
- **Demonstrate a variety of pose variations.** Often students will emulate what you are doing, so when you demonstrate, don't default to the

most complex variation of the pose. Demonstrate within a range of motion accessible to the students in front of you.

- **Explain what you are doing and why.** Avoid saying a pose will make you feel X, Y, Z or explaining poses in terms of their goals. Instead, give the option for your students to tune in to sensations of spaciousness, resistance, and awareness of the space around them. For trauma survivors the experience and ability of being connected to their bodies will likely be complex – so keep everything optional, including tuning in to physical sensations.

- **Emphasize the space around your students.** Yoga often focuses on interoceptive experiences (an awareness of sensations inside the body), but emphasizing proprioception is helpful for many students, particularly survivors. Proprioception is an awareness of where our bodies are in space. This might mean feeling your feet press into the mat, the sensation of your fingers extending upwards, using props, and exploring poses at the wall. Proprioceptive awareness gives an alternative way to acknowledge your body and spend time with it without dwelling on internal sensations.

- **Be authentic.** Let go of the performance of yourself as a perfect/zen/aligned teacher. If you make a mistake, acknowledge it and laugh about it. If you are injured and restricted in how you are practising, say so. Students will trust your humanity more than a performance of authority.

- **Verbally recognize and celebrate the variety of choices your students take.** Be mindful that students may not be comfortable being individually pointed out (unless that rapport has been established between you over time), but acknowledge the variety of great choices you see in the room.

- **Model props and lay them out beforehand.** Many students may not feel confident reaching for props or know what they might need in advance.

- **Get to know your students and their communication style.** Teach in a way that supports students with different communication needs and be willing to explain a pose in multiple ways.

- **Avoid prescriptive breathing patterns.** Simply encouraging your students to breathe is enough, especially if you notice them holding their breaths. If you do teach a specific class style where you offer movements cued with the inhale or exhale, keep the breathing invitational and make sure students know they can (and should) take extra breaths as needed.

- **Adjustments: in general, and in a specified trauma-aware class, steer clear of hands-on adjustments.** If you do offer adjustments, make them your last resort, and make sure that you state in your class description that consensual adjustments are offered. Keep reconfirming consent; receiving consent at the start of class is not enough alone. As the teacher, it is your responsibility to actively foster an environment where changing your mind is celebrated.
- **Find a rhythm.** Don't be afraid of repetition; it can be soothing and reassuring. Improving self-regulation takes time and repetition is essential for this. We can use repetition in the way we use our voice, and in our directions, affirmations, and movement patterns. Allow rhythmicity to be a part of your class. Flow, pause, flow, pause to allow for stimulating and soothing the nervous system.
- **Ground in environment.** Offer regular opportunities to orientate to the environment by cueing the students' attention to sounds, light, physical sensations, and even smells.

THE EXISTING TRAUMA TRAINING CULTURE

At the risk of kicking the hornets' nest, the current trauma-informed teaching and training culture desperately needs some critical evaluation. Although this isn't true of all trainings (or teachers), many of them – including some of the most established ones – overlook some fundamental elements of trauma survivors' experiences. Consequently, they have developed teaching modalities that are ineffective or unsafe for many trauma survivors. 'Trauma-aware' and 'trauma-informed' have become catch-all phrases in yoga spaces. However, if you are looking to develop or undertake trauma-informed trainings, we have four important questions for you to consider.

Who developed or who is teaching the trauma-informed yoga courses?

Most often, the answer is not trauma survivors. Trauma-informed trainings are frequently developed from a top-down perspective instead of built from the bottom up. These courses rely on what the existing research and theories say, and are full of generalizations about what trauma is and how to navigate it and potentially 'heal' from it in a yoga setting. Many courses and practitioners are well intentioned, but often they are misinformed because they don't have the relevant lived experience. This also opens up important conversations about who is profiting from the hard-won experience of trauma survivors.

How does the course think about and define trauma?

Trauma is as old as humanity itself, but as a diagnosed medical condition, it is an incredibly young phenomenon, as discussed by Amelia Wood in the preceding chapter. There are a growing number of conditions that relate to trauma. This is all positive. However, it is likely this is just the tip of the iceberg. Much trauma is self-diagnosed. For many people, particularly those who face systemic discrimination, seeking help or a diagnosis based on their trauma can be a traumatic experience in and of itself. There is a high probability that they will be misdiagnosed and receive incorrect treatment. The medical and scientific insights on trauma are not redundant. However, they are not the be-all and end-all. Nor should they take precedence over a survivor's reported experience. If a trauma-informed course is only rooted in research and evidence-based approaches, it will most often be placing the scientific community's understanding of trauma over that of the survivors.

How is trauma-informed yoga taught?

Given that trauma and its fallouts are so wildly complex, how is it possible to teach in a trauma-sensitive and safe way? Frequently, trauma-informed teacher trainings consist of a checklist of things to do and not do, teach and not teach, say and not say. This is built upon a rigorous, although probably simplified, understanding of the trauma response and nervous system regulation. There is scientific theory, with a teaching theory layered on top, and a checklist on how to enforce that theory on top of that. All these theories and checklists have somehow been shown to be effective and true for the cohorts that have been studied. On top of this, some trauma-informed classes will claim to heal trauma and promise to be trigger-free. Given the themes we have discussed in this chapter so far, we hope all this is causing you to raise an eyebrow.

As we have said before, everything about trauma is complex. If you are promising a trauma-informed class and one in every five students is falling through the cracks of what you are selling, surely we have an issue. To give just one example, many trauma-informed courses advocate the use of specific breathing patterns and ratios, including 'coherent breathing', which involves bringing awareness to your breathing and slowing it down. This is troubling for several reasons:

- Consciously being aware of and slowing the breath down can be a trigger.
- The evidence-based rationale for this system stems from one very small-scale and not particularly high-quality study on the use of coherent breathing with Iyengar yoga for 15 people with depressive

disorders, most of whom had experience with trauma.[3] The exclusion criteria for this study included anyone who was in psychotherapy, on medication, 'overweight', who consumed alcohol, or had experienced suicidal thoughts, amongst other criteria.

- Although different variations of coherent breathing are taught, the practice is trademarked by someone who claims to have invented the breathing practice. The cultural appropriation of yoga practices by some scientists claiming to have invented *prāṇāyāma* practices is a common and deeply problematic issue.

The effects of any breath practice can be unpredictable, and whilst there is the potential for them to be supportive, freeing, and nurturing there is just as much possibility that they can be overwhelming, over-activating, or even terror- and panic-inducing. There is no panacea, no definitive breathwork that works for everyone. And so, as with all our offerings, our role as teacher is to go gently, understand the likely result of a practice, and at the same time hold the possibility that it may be very different for the people in front of us.

Who is selling you your training?

Like many other areas of yoga, the rise of trauma-informed yoga is at a comfortable intersection with capitalism and the multi-billion-dollar wellness industry. There has been a spike in trauma-informed trainings and classes recently. At its most insidious (and yoga can be very insidious), trainings have been developed in response to market demand, effectively capitalizing on trauma.

We would encourage you to thoroughly research any training related to trauma that you would be interested in undertaking. Look for trainings that are person-centred, community-focused, rooted in social justice, non-dogmatic, and critically aware. Given the ideas we have highlighted above for making your teaching safer for those who have experienced trauma, you might take a look at the training and critically evaluate whether they are using these principles themselves in how they represent, market, and sell the course. Lastly, take a look at how their pricing is structured: do they offer bursaries for marginalized populations?

WHAT IS A YOGA TEACHER'S RESPONSIBILITY?

You may be relieved to read we are here to absolve you of (some of) these perceived responsibilities as a trauma-informed yoga teacher. You should have a very specific code of conduct and duty to your students as a yoga teacher.

However, regardless of how much training, research, or personal experience of trauma you have, you are not a therapist or trauma specialist in the context of teaching a yoga class. You are a yoga teacher. How the yoga class space is navigated differs from how therapeutic and treatment spaces are conducted.

Respecting the boundaries of your role as a yoga teacher is essential for both you and your students. Even if you think you might be able to help a student in some way that transgresses the boundaries of the yoga space, don't. Your student did not consent to that and you don't know how quickly you might get out of your depth and unwittingly cause harm.

Your students might also appeal to you for support that extends beyond what you are capable of as a yoga teacher. If so, you have options: you can signpost them on to other helpful resources; having a network of charities, therapists, physios, and other professionals that you can *personally vouch for* is incredibly helpful as a teacher. If you don't have a suitable person or organization to recommend, then acknowledge that and say that what they are asking is beyond your scope. If they find your classes helpful, they are welcome to keep coming, and signpost them towards fields and modalities you have an understanding of that may be helpful.

Doing something that transgresses your role as a yoga teacher is an abuse of power. You may not feel that it is, and it may be a small abuse compared to the ones we are so used to reading about in the media, but it is an abuse of power nonetheless.

If on the other hand a student is in distress, simply treat them as you would any other person that is in distress. Ask what they need or if there is someone you can call, just as if a student was bleeding or had injured themself in your class. The key is to create a space where students feel safe enough to verbalize and take action about what they need.

Holding hope

For people affected by trauma, yoga is by no means the cure-all it's portrayed to be. However, its regulatory nature can be of help to manage some of the stress-related symptoms that arise. The potential for positive outcomes through a regular yoga practice is undeniable. But the reality is that for many people, working through their trauma responses in a way that is respectful, empowering, and safe is extremely difficult. As teachers we mustn't fall into the trap of thinking we need to see radical change in our students. Rather we can become the holders of hope, holding the possibility of change without any attachment or expectation. And perhaps, sometimes, for some people, positive change can happen as a result.

ON SURVIVING

Theo Wildcroft and Harriet McAtee

For our final chapter in this section, once again we wanted to include a more personal reflection on the theme of trauma. We, Harriet and Theo, are both survivors of long-term, interpersonal abuse. This is sometimes given the clinical label of 'complex trauma' or even 'treatment-resistant trauma'.

What we know for certain is that conversations about trauma between survivors are very different to conversations with non-survivors. There is a common ground, not of experience, but of tone: a familiarity with dark humour and complex emotions, an understanding that the world is home to both more pain and more joy than many people realize.

For this chapter, then, Theo and Harriet recorded a conversation on our experiences as survivors teaching and practising yoga. Together, we explore such themes as: perceptions of time and healing, being a 'good survivor' and the fatigue of survivorship, the fallacy of 'completion' in healing, the holistic and interconnected impact of trauma on a survivor's life, the mundanity of practice versus the drama of performance, the dangers of prioritizing the practice over the person, the co-existence of joy and suffering, and the reality of being both broken and healed at the same time.

Whilst this chapter does not contain references to specific incidents, a content note for the general themes of abuse and trauma still applies.

Theo

One of the things I wanted to recognize as we begin is the positionality of being a teacher, and a trainer, and a survivor.

I get frustrated by how unforgiving people are of process and time in survivorship. Yet over time, my understanding of that has changed. Early on in my life, I needed to believe that there would be an end point to healing where everything would be okay, and I wouldn't have to deal with this any more. I think I wouldn't have been able to contemplate then the idea of living with this for the rest of my life – the injustice of that fact, and the huge lack of support on that journey.

It's not just that you didn't choose this trauma and it was caused in many cases by situations or organizations and people that hold no accountability for what they've done. It's also that there's not really much support. There's that terrible phrase 'treatment-resistant complex PTSD'. So, if you can even get a kind of diagnosis or at least recognition that you need help, that help is so often so inadequate.

I don't think I'd have been able to tell my 21-year-old self, 'You will be dealing with this the rest of your life. And pretty much the only significant support you will reliably get along the way will be from other survivors. Places that you will go for healing will be a lottery. Some of those places will re-traumatize you. And there is no justice.'

I am, in so many ways, stronger than I've ever been, more self-aware than I've ever been, and more able to navigate my life than I could ever have imagined. But it's hard. And sometimes you are just tired of it. If I could wrap this up and put it away for a bit, I would.

Harriet

I really hear that. I think it's really interesting, particularly when it comes to teaching and practising yoga, where we work with students who might be very goal-oriented. A really big part of my healing (although I don't like that word), a really big part of my process, has been integration. (That is a word I like.) It means working with how I integrate these experiences that I had, which were traumatic and challenging and painful, so that I can understand them in the context of my life.

And one of the things that has been really important to me in that process of integration is letting go almost entirely of the idea of goal setting. It's not something I do really in any area of my life.

I think that's an interesting thing in the context of people approaching yoga as a practice to help them process, heal, or manage trauma: the intention or the framework that you bring to the practice in those instances becomes so crucial because if it's about fixing or neutralizing trauma somehow, you're setting yourself up for disappointment.

And as you say, the people who I have found the most support around are other survivors.

Theo

I think we also need to recognize that the other issue with goal setting is it doesn't recognize how interconnected everything is. When I say I'll live with this for the rest of my life, I guess people who don't understand survivorship and trauma think that means living with daily triggers and panic attacks and so on. And it's not. It's living with random dysphoria. It's not having parental support in times of financial need. It's completely holistic in its impact on my life. It affects how I navigate relationships in ways I can't disentangle.

And some of that can be really positive. Post-traumatic growth is real. But again, we think about post-traumatic growth as being something different from ongoing post-traumatic conditions. And for me, they're the same thing. What has made it more possible for me to manage my symptoms over time more than anything is my changing and evolving awareness of the interconnectedness of my situation. It's another layer of my identity, just like coming out, or my neurodivergence. The route of my understanding of both of those things too was completely inflected by my family history and experiences.

That's why when I was 16, I wasn't able to consider being queer because I was so invested in the idea of being 'normal', because I was so invested in the idea that what had happened to me wouldn't fundamentally change me. I would have come out much earlier without that. And in a similar way, in the last year I've moved from thinking of myself as primarily a survivor who is neurodivergent, to starting to contemplate the ways in which my neurodivergence has made me more isolated and vulnerable and more of a target for predators.

There are all sorts of marginalization. And social marginalization makes us more vulnerable to suffering so many different kinds of trauma.

So, these things are complex. They're societal. And they're structural. The reason why people want survivors to only exist as totally healed or totally broken (and under medical care) is partly because they don't want to look at the systemic nature of trauma within our social systems and our interpersonal dynamics. They don't want to feel the magnitude of that ongoing pain and injustice.

Harriet

My experience of talking about my history and my trauma, my process, is that there's a lot of fear in that for me. Because you open yourself up to understanding and seeing trauma on a societal level, on top of your own individual experience.

Every time I unpack a little bit more of myself, I become more integrated and my understanding grows. As you say, in so many ways, the way I relate to people and myself and the world is affected by my trauma. Every time I discover something new in it, or see it in a new way, there's a relief – suddenly I understand myself better. But there's also a real grieving happening for me, not only for my own experiences but also for what's happening more broadly in the world. And it's so tiring.

Theo

I do think yoga can give us the tools to reflect on this in ways that are helpful. And hopefully that allows us to understand other people's traumas. I'm aware, for example, of my internal resistance as a white person to really taking on board the reality of ongoing racial trauma, rather than events that happened 50 years ago or more. You can intellectually understand that these injustices are ongoing. But to really understand the ongoing impact of microaggressions and structural issues around marginalized identities is different.

Harriet

It's like trying to talk to any man about the experience of being femme. I love men but they cannot really understand a world in which you could get in an elevator and be brutally aware of the fact that you're the only woman in there and be scared by that.

Theo

I was going to say that the mundane nature of it is really important. We don't need to talk about our personal, individual histories of trauma because what happened to me is banal in its everydayness. And yet if I open up to people about it, they say, 'Oh my God, that's terrible.' It becomes dramatic. But in my case, you could literally write a case study of the most typical pattern of child sexual abuse and my history ticks every box.

It's terrible, but what we go through is also mundane. That kind of trauma and so many others, it's around us all the time. And it's a mark of such privilege not to know that, to see it as something strange and terrible that needs urgent care, rather than the default history of so much of humanity.

Harriet

Maybe this is going to be an unpopular opinion, but there's a mundaneness to yoga practice as well. Not in the sense that it's boring, but there's a lot of repetition.

And one of the things I'm really interested in, that I think is one of the most useful aspects of yoga, is seeing your practice as a microcosm of the world at large. Your practice is a platform or a medium through which you get to rehearse agency, and you get to rehearse consent, and you get to rehearse bodily strength.

Anyone who has to rehearse or learn a piece of music or other performance – it's an art form, there's a peak moment, but there's also a mundaneness to how you arrive at that outcome or how you come into that experience of performing, you know?

Theo

I think you're right. We conflate the practice with the performance in yoga. With those kinds of embodied skills, as dramatic or spectacular as that performance is, the actual practice of it is mundane, and even boring and repetitive and annoying at times.

Maybe there's something that's happened with workshop culture in yoga, where we feel like every encounter between yoga teacher and student has to be a performance rather than a practice? So it's all: ' Wow I have never been able to touch my toes and I just touched my toes. And now you have healed my life in a way I've never been healed before.' Rather than 'Okay, it's Wednesday, let's see if we can touch our toes today. And maybe we'll get further than we did last week, and maybe we won't.'

The mundaneness of it, and a commitment to that, is important for both students and teachers. And you're right. I think if there's one thing that I would want to change about teaching survivors, it's that I want teachers to know that what is happening is mundane and everyday for me.

You're not here to heal me. I'm not going to walk in as if it's an evangelical church, and the power of the gods is not flowing through your teaching space whilst I breathe and move. It's Wednesday and I am just seeing if I can unpeel another layer and feel a little freer today.

Harriet

I think one of the things I am very sure about, in my teaching and in the work that I do, is how much I don't want to take over the world.

Despite the fact that we're writing a book that will presumably be read by quite a few people, I'm not actually really interested in attaining a high level of success or acclaim. I have quite modest ambitions. Important for me as well is the responsibility that comes along with our role as practitioners and teachers.

I have moments of performance, of course, because they're required of us to be able to teach. But I'm not interested in the performance. I'm interested in how practice, and the everydayness of it, the mundaneness, is able to support me in integrating further.

Theo

Yeah. I think that also that attitude of performance gets in the way of what yoga teachers need to do with students. It feeds into the idea that the yoga teacher must be the expert with the magic solution.

I say this a lot, but the number of Facebook threads you see with yoga teachers saying, 'I have a student with this condition, can they do this? Can they do that? How am I going to help them?' And I always want to say, 'Have you asked them?'

When I've worked with disabled people, very often, I haven't had a clear or expert understanding of their conditions because each condition can be rare and unusual. In the end, all you can say is 'Okay, what can they do? What can they not do? What do they enjoy? What would help them live with a little more ease?' And when you do that, rather than thinking it's a syndrome characterized by a lack of collagen fibres or whatever, what you actually get is useful answers, such as: their digestion isn't great, so can we work on something that might help that today? Or this person has trouble tying their shoelaces and that gives them anxiety, is there something we can do to help with hand coordination today?

That's why I think yoga teaching is much more aligned to that idea of occupational health – that there are tasks that you need to do in order to thrive as a human being. The everyday tasks are what are important, not whether you can run a marathon or put your legs behind your head. We really need to bring that into the heart of yoga teaching. Until we do that, I don't think we'll be properly serving many of our students.

And that will also stop us effectively reconciling with the reality of trauma in our classes, because these supposedly extraordinary conditions are actually really mundane, and the solutions people need are individual and based in their own habits and practices.

You need to really talk to people to find out not what they've suffered, or even what diagnosis they were able to get, but how their trauma shows up for them, and what they already know. I guarantee that anyone you're going to have as a yoga student already knows a lot about how to manage their daily life, unless you're working in a secure unit somewhere.

I think it's very similar to the fear of 'bad' alignment that teachers have sometimes, where they say, 'If you're going to bend over safely, you must do it exactly this way.' You realize people bend over all the time, right? They haven't died from it yet.

Harriet

I think to put what you're saying another way, what we need is a student-centred approach to the teaching and practice of yoga. Not putting teachers on pedestals is important, and I think we've already gone a little way with that in the contemporary yoga landscape.

But where I see the biggest issue, which is much more insidious, is in putting the practice on a pedestal. I see lots of yoga teachers doing it, and that's the bit I get really concerned about. There are lots of teachers who will think that they're being really inclusive and accessible, and they are well intentioned. And they might have done some thinking about de-emphasizing the role of the teacher, or they might believe that they work really collaboratively. But the yoga, or the practice, is still the thing that they're prioritizing over their students, over the people in front of them.

In my experience when yoga teachers get this distinction, they really get it, but it can be a subtle and trickier thing for teachers to achieve. Because if you let go of the role of the practice as being at the centre of the teaching, then you start to ask yourself, 'Well, what am I doing?' You know?

Theo

Yes. You have to be comfortable suggesting to people that maybe what they really need is a nice long walk every morning, or a martial arts practice, rather than more sun salutations.

What my 'practice' actually is changes and evolves. By no means all of it looks like yoga. And certainly, since the pandemic started, a lot of it has looked like walking, because I've needed to move, I've needed to travel through space, not stay on my mat. And I know I'm not the only yoga teacher that's found this.

Now, on the one hand, yoga teachers are really good at saying, 'Oh, everything is yoga', but at the same time, we can still be trapped by the mat, right? A truly inclusive and open practice would say, 'Well, how are you using all possible tools for your self-care?' And 'How are you using the wisdom you already have?'

Because if a new student doesn't already have a yoga practice that we recognize as such, we treat them as someone who doesn't know anything about self-care for their condition. Whereas the sensible thing to say to someone who's been living with any kind of long-term, chronic condition is 'What do you already know? What already works for you?' And then if someone replies, 'Well, you know, Pilates really helps my lower back', then okay, great. That tells me something about what works for you already.

Harriet

Yeah, 100 per cent. I think it's going to be interesting to see what the next five or ten years hold in terms of how the practice evolves and responds to accessible, student-centred approaches to teaching.

To echo what you're saying, my practice also changes all the time. And one of my teachers talks about the idea of 'stupid compassion', which I love. This is the idea that you can be compassionate and you can love, but if you're not critical enough of what the actual impact of that is, or what the cost of that is to you, then that is stupid compassion and it can harm more than help. So, a really classic example would be really giving to others at the expense of your own energy.

And he also talks about stupid meditation, which is really lovely. I do stupid meditation all the time, where I just sit and I look like I'm meditating but really, I'm just off in another world and there's nothing being cultivated there.

I wonder if maybe a lot of the practice that people do is just stupid practice. Not in the sense that it's harmful, but it's woolly. It's a displacement activity. Which is necessary sometimes. Displacement activities have a real role to play. But it's almost like busy work.

Theo

There's also a strong link between the busy work of practice and the ritualization of a defence mechanism that says, 'If I do this then I will not get sick, no one in my family will die, and my relationships will work out, and I will not have to deal with loss and grief – and trauma.'

Suffering is real, and so is joy. We are all of these things. And yoga can help. But when I'm playful with a group of students, and especially when we're playing around with something quite challenging and they get very involved, one of my favourite things to do is remind them in that moment that nothing they are doing will stop them from getting old, sick, or dying. And then usually they laugh and fall out of whatever we're doing.

I think it's a really important thing to remember. Because otherwise this practice is just a ritualized sort of defence theatre. Nothing we're doing is going to change the fact that one day, something is going to hurt. You can't stop that happening. And that doesn't mean you need to be in a place of grief and suffering all the time. It doesn't mean not to feel joy.

And as a survivor, I think that's the other lesson that we can embody for other people – that inasmuch as our conditions will never go away, and inasmuch as there is no justice, it does not change the profound joy and pleasure that we are still able to have in our lives. Our experiences run the full range. We live in a kind of technicolour where those things can co-exist and do co-occur in each and every day. And it's in our human capacity to be all of those things. And the practice of yoga can help us hold that and manage it well, rather than just to hold on tight to only the moments of joy.

Harriet

Definitely. And that brings us back nicely to where we started, talking about those two images or models of survivorship – the broken and the healed. When the reality is, we are not one or the other, we're both.

Theo

Yeah. Both of those realities – brokenness and healing – exist in all survivors each and every day. That's a nice place to stop. Quite poetically.

RACE. JUSTICE. EQUITY.

12 —

INTRODUCING OMWASHING

Sheena Sood

Sheena has been practising yoga since she was 13 years old. Her early visits to India consisted of her learning mantras from her grandmother, Biji. As she learned about how Brahmins and Hindu nationalists were weaponizing yoga to advance divisive and oppressive agendas across the South Asian region and the world, she became uncertain if she could trust her yoga practice to hold space for the social justice values she strived to embody.

But when she moved to Philadelphia to begin a doctoral pro-gramme at Temple University, she yearned for a spiritual routine that anchored her in synchronized movement with the breath and connected her to her ancestors. So in between studying, she travelled to the Himalayas to become certified as an advanced yoga practitioner with Yogi Sivadas at the Kailash Tribal School.

Today, Sheena's research as a social scientist scrutinizes the oppressive arms of the yoga industry. At the same time, she works with adults, children, collectives, and organizations to help them incor-porate spiritual traditions (like yoga and meditation), holistic health wisdom, and wellness practices into their lives. She believes (as do we) that in order for healing traditions to support people's capacity to evolve and support collective freedom struggles, they must be offered and embodied through a politicized lens, and that spiritual teachers and entrepreneurs must be critical of the ways these practices have been co-opted and weaponized for oppressive agendas.

For this chapter, Sheena has gifted us with a much-needed refram-ing of yoga and cultural appropriation, through the lens of orientalism. This is a vital critique of the current mainstream solutions, which weaponize identity politics and all too often reinforce racial capitalism, caste-based oppression, and far-right ethnonationalism. She does this through three key examples: the use of Sanskrit in contemporary yoga settings; yoga teaching in prisons; and the celebration of International Yoga Day. Sheena calls for yoga to be rooted in liberation theology, allied with international solidarity and abolitionism.

THE ASSUMPTIONS OF AUM

The first time I recall hearing Sanskrit, I was visiting my grandmother in India. Biji taught me chants like the *Gayatri Mantra*. She offered me a glimpse into reconnecting with my ancestral traditions.

My entry point to a formal study of Sanskrit came while I was completing my yoga teacher training at Kailash Tribal School in McLeodganj, India. My guru, Yogi Sivadas, emphasized the sacred origins of Sanskrit. He shared that the mantra *om* (or *aum*) in particular is considered to be a primordial sound – one that was heard before the universe even came into formation: 'Before there was "om," there was nothing.'

It is not uncommon for yogis across the globe to remark on the sacredness of *aum*. Both through my familial and cultural networks, and through my study of yoga, the narrative I have heard is that *aum* is a universally auspicious mantra that operates on an especially high vibration. When we chant *aum*, we elevate our consciousness. Accordingly, I have used Sanskrit mantras for healing rituals for myself and in the yoga classes I teach.

In recent years, however, I have been more reluctant to chant and use Sanskrit in personal and collective yoga spaces – especially as I consider the pain and oppression that Sanskrit and Hinduism have long inflicted on marginalized communities in the South Asian region.

I have written in previous publications about how elite Brahmanical groups in pre-colonial South Asia reserved the use of Sanskrit mantras for upper-caste networks to maintain economic and political dominance in the region.[1] Brahmin priests and scholars chanted Sanskrit for their own spiritual ceremonies and rituals, but they violently punished marginalized castes for merely being in the presence of Sanskrit.

While I understand mantras and sound vibration to have a powerful cleansing effect throughout the various circuits of the body, the more I study the dynamics of power and oppression in South Asian society, the more I am invited to a space of critical wonder. For instance, when yogis proclaim that *aum* is a universally divine mantra, I wonder whether they question how this understanding has been constructed through a casteist lens. One of the reasons we are told that *aum* operates on such a high vibrational frequency is because it represents *Brahman* – the deity associated with creation. Brahmin is also regarded as the highest category by the socio-religious hierarchy known as the varna or caste system. I can't help but wonder, is *aum* considered to be a universally healing mantra because of its energetic vibration, or because Brahmins proclaim it to be so?

I don't think yoga students and practitioners generally question the dominant narratives supplanted by Brahmanical Hindu culture. After all, yoga certification programs in the West, and also in the East, circulate the romanticized narrative that assumes *aum* to be an inherently positive mantra. But we should. We should question and critically challenge them as well.

As a yoga teacher, *I am expected to know, share, and reproduce the romanticized narrative* associated with *aum*, the one that emphasizes how chanting Sanskrit automatically connects us to a higher vibrational healing power. *I am not, however, expected to complicate this narrative* by entertaining the counternarratives proposed by marginalized Desi communities – the ones that associate Sanskrit with violence, hierarchy, and oppression.

I find this to be a dangerous tendency.

As a sociologist who studies the history of yoga's continuous appropriation by the West *and* by the East, I have observed whites and South Asians be equally complicit in disseminating a monolithic yogic narrative that locks Sanskrit (and yoga) in a glorified past. The former narratives erase the contributions of Desis to yogic culture while the latter narratives falsely attribute ownership to Hindu elites in the South Asian region. Part of how these singular narratives are perpetuated is embedded in the legacy of colonialism and the framework of *orientalism*.

THE LEGACY OF EDWARD SAID'S *ORIENTALISM* ON YOGIC CULTURE

Orientalism as a Western style for dominating, restructuring, and having authority over the Orient... Without examining Orientalism as a discourse one cannot possibly understand the enormously systematic discipline by which European culture was able to manage – and even produce – the Orient politically, sociologically, militarily, ideologically, scientifically, and imaginatively during the post-Enlightenment period.[2]

The tendency to romanticize Sanskrit as a universally healing language and yogic culture as an inherently pure and peaceful spiritual tradition is embedded in a colonial legacy of how Western culture has sought to represent – or rather *misrepresent* – the East.

Edward Said, the late cultural critic and philosopher, first coined the theoretical framework of 'orientalism' in 1974. Embedded in his theory is the argument that the framing of the East by the West can be understood through the imperial logic of '*orientalism*', a discourse that stereotypes the 'orient' as *timeless* and *spiritually rich* – as opposed to *scientific* and *logical*. *Orientalism* is a critique of modern European colonialism and imperialism. It sees colonialism not only as a brutal and exploitative system of political rule, but also as a worldview that conditions the Western gaze toward the East.

'Orientalism' continues to find relevance and application to contemporary imaginings of the East. It conditions people who study and become immersed in Eastern cultures to uncritically revere and accept ancient and mystical wisdom as objective truth.

Within the yoga world, the absence of critical thinking is dangerous for a number of reasons.

First, orientalism lends itself to a tendency to lock South Asian history, the cultural birthplace of yoga, in a time capsule that does not engage with the inevitability of evolutionary change.

Consider the claim that 'yoga is a 5000-year-old tradition'.

In the popular imagination, claims like this presume yoga to have an unbroken lineage. Yet, these claims do not reflect historical reality – a reality that emphasizes yoga's *constant change* according to social and political contexts.

Second, Said also writes, 'My hope is to illustrate the formidable structure of cultural domination and, specifically for formerly colonized peoples, the dangers and temptations of employing the structure upon themselves.'[3] The concern with South Asians internalizing orientalist logic with respect to yoga is that when internalized, *orientalism* lends itself to a type of identity politics – one that flattens the identity of formerly colonized people whose culture is being represented.

In an attempt to confront the power dynamics and cultural appropriation of yoga in contemporary spiritual spaces, which are informed by colonial and white supremacist logics, yogis of color – many of them Desi (or South Asian) – suggest that the solutions to the erasure of people of color in yoga spaces are to: (1) train more Black and Indigenous people of color (BIPOC) teachers; (2) diversify yoga spaces; (3) listen to South Asian yoga teachers; and

(4) honor yoga's roots (which are assumed to have an ancient, authentic, and pure origin story). In other words, these solutions advocate for more diversity and representation of Brown people as solutions to the marginalization and erasure of South Asians from mainstream yoga spaces. But the idea of yoga as having a monolithic past is reified in these solutions.

Although yogic philosophy invites us to surrender to the wisdom that change is inevitable, there is a tendency to lock yoga history itself in a static past. Those in the East and the West internalize the representation of Eastern culture as a fixed essence in their attempt to resolve issues of cultural appropriation.

While I understand that these solutions, which are couched in the rhetoric of 'cultural appropriation' and 'decolonization', stem from the erasure of South Asian faces in yoga spaces, my fear is that such solutions further weaponize identity politics toward advancing racial capitalism, caste-based oppression, and Hindu fundamentalism.

As a result, the South Asian voices that are leveraged to speak about yoga's 'ancient' and 'traditional' past often refuse to acknowledge the embeddedness of yogic culture in a casteist and religious fundamentalist context. They are more attuned to the optics of representation in yoga spaces than they are to the ethics of where and how yoga is being deployed.

Finally, these voices often assume yoga to be rooted in a socially just past, a past that assumes power and oppression played no part in how that philosophy was interpreted and shared across time, space, and history.

The framework of orientalism continues to operate as a weapon of imperialist logic today; the only difference is that the perpetrators of colonial and imperial logics are not simply of the West; they are of the East as well.

ORIENTALISM AT WORK: CONTEMPORARY EXOTIFICATIONS OF YOGA AS PURE

We also assume as yoga teachers that the ways in which yoga is couched in contemporary structures and social institutions are inherently for the greater good. The exotification of yoga as pure and inherently beneficial or healing to all people who have an opportunity to practice it is a contemporary manifestation of the same orientalism at work.

Again, rather than being concerned with matters of *representation* in yoga spaces, yoga teachers ought to be more concerned with the *ethics* of *how and for what purpose* yoga is deployed to various populations. Allow me to explain my argument using two case studies, one that analyzes yoga's use in prisons and another that analyzes the global popularity of International Day of Yoga.

CASE STUDY 1: YOGA IN PRISONS

I've worked here for five years now. The youth here get into a lot of fights. They're dealing with pent-up anger and acting on pain, and they're in a place where their movement is restricted. After all I've witnessed working on the inside, I know for sure there is no law I would break that would send me to jail. That's why I try to show these kids that though they think they got it bad on the outside, it isn't *as bad* as the inside. So, whatever they're thinking about doing, think again, it isn't worth it. That's why the yoga work you do with them is so important. Anything that teaches them to foster inner peace, so they can *behave* better and learn self-control so they don't end up back here is helpful, if they know how to value it.

Anonymous juvenile justice services center staff member[4]

In January of 2020, I started teaching a weekly trauma-informed mindfulness and yoga session in the young women's unit at a local juvenile justice services center. While I am an abolitionist who believes in fighting for a world where prisons, walls, and borders do not exist, I teach yoga inside an institution that cages youth because penitentiaries are such a pervasive and normalized part of American society. Although youth and adults in the carceral system are discouraged from feeling a sense of connection with their bodies, their health, and overall humanity, I believe they have the right to (re)connect to a quality of oneness within themselves. I agreed to offer yoga in prisons in the hopes that incarcerated youth and adults would be able to find a momentary sense of awareness of their own humanity and capacity for love and transformation.

Yoga practitioners bring a range of beliefs and ethics to their programs in prisons. In the epigraph above, the juvenile justice services center staff member saw my yoga program as a valuable asset to the prison's recreational program, because he felt it would help the youth reform their behavior and make 'smarter' decisions. He assumes such behavioral shifts could result in these youth not getting arrested or caught up in the (penal) system. Through improving their attitudes, the staff member implied that guards (or law enforcement officers) would not 'be forced' to use violence to constrain them in 'tough situations'. The staff member's logic fits with the common belief that *the justice system can be reformed* and that the onus is on those who are held captive in the system to rehabilitate themselves within it.

Recently, I was watching a Netflix miniseries called *The Mind, Explained*, specifically the episode on 'Mindfulness'.[5] Generally, I was impressed with the episode's capacity to break down the positive impact of mindfulness meditation on the brain. A portion of the episode discussed the capacity of mindfulness to help practitioners rewire and create new pathways of communicating with the brain.

Still, I couldn't help but notice that the conversation on mindfulness and yoga was devoid of an analysis of the broader racial and economic landscape. Featuring the example of sharing yoga with prisoners in the John Moran Medium Security Facility in Cranston, Rhode Island, a mindfulness teacher expressed how meditation serves as a training ground for developing a healthy mind. She explains, 'How can you have something happen and create enough emotional space to make a choice that isn't the reaction that's going to get them into trouble over and over again? Can I be aware of myself? Can I manage what's happening inside of me so *I can manage my behaviour*? The possibility is to start to create a different version of themselves.'[6]

Couched within this instructor's words is the assumption that the problem is with the prisoners' behavior, not with the system of incarceration itself. Absent from the dialogue is a structural and racialized critique around prisons. And prison yoga is not an uncommon phenomenon. Before COVID-19, prison yoga programs were booming across the US.

The prison yoga example illustrates how the discourse of orientalism pervades the perception and circulation of yoga. While the instructors of prison yoga programs are likely well-meaning teachers who want to share breathing and mindfulness techniques with individuals who have limited access to such resources, such programs use yoga and spirituality to divert attention away from the inherent structural violence of their institutions. This is what I call 'omwashing'. Rather than demanding change and putting political pressure on the system to transform or restructure the system of policing and mass incarceration to be less racist and classist, these programs cooperate quite neatly with a racist, classist system.

Can we see how the emphasis here on a solution that assumes yoga to be a pure and peaceful tradition that will automatically bring good things to incarcerated people rests on orientalist logics? It is based on two assumptions: that bringing yoga to people who are otherwise not represented in yoga is inherently good for them, and that the criminal justice system is just. They lead to the conclusion that a prisoner learning how to achieve inner peace and/or enlightenment is going to lead to radical and revolutionary change, when the reality is that such programs do not make a radical dent in the processes of mass incarceration.

We need yoga teachers in prisons who understand the depth of structural violence affecting poor communities of color, which renders them vulnerable to high incarceration rates. We need teachers who recognize prisons as inhumane, oppressive systems, instructors who are committed to tearing down the systems that cage poor Black and Brown bodies, and who see spiritual liberation as an internal and external process and pathway to transformation.

There are some major distinctions between those who believe the prison system can be *reformed* versus those who believe it needs to be completely *abolished*. Those in the reformist camp hope to improve conditions inside prisons, while those in abolitionist movements object to the existence of prisons altogether. Abolitionists seek to replace the 'justice' system's punitive models with more transformative systems of accountability and harm reduction. Abolitionists believe that the pathway to eradicating harm/injustice must happen through getting at the root causes of violence.

In order for yoga to be an effective tool for spiritual, mental, emotional, and physical liberation, it needs to be couched in an *abolitionist* – rather than a reformist (and neoliberal) – political framework. While the pairing of yoga with an abolitionist lens is not limited to prison-based yoga offerings, an abolitionist approach to integrating yoga programs in the prison system can serve as a model for how yoga is practiced and shared outside these spaces. Working from an abolitionist lens allows us to start from a space of full freedom, rather than one of partial freedom, and it anchors the teaching of yoga in an ethics that validates humanity and the right to liberation for all people.

CASE STUDY 2: INTERNATIONAL DAY OF YOGA

One of the most widely celebrated yoga holidays across the globe is International Day of Yoga, which takes place on June 21 and coincides with the summer (or winter) solstice each year. The largest yoga class on record, which gathered over 100,000 participants in Kota, Rajasthan, was held in 2018 in honor of International Yoga Day.

The holiday's popularity is also underscored by the over 600,000 social media users on Instagram who have used the hashtags #InternationalDayOfYoga or #InternationalYogaDay to draw attention to the ways that yoga has shaped and transformed their lives. In recent years, even during the height of the COVID-19 pandemic, yoga studios, teachers, and organizations around the globe have insisted on capitalizing on the momentum of the holiday to spread awareness about the benefits that a regular yoga practice brings to their lives. From places like New York City to Dublin to New Delhi to Athens to Kyiv, people have organized free public yoga classes.

Although yoga itself is popularly celebrated as a timeless tradition, International Day of Yoga is actually quite a young holiday. It was initiated in 2014, after Prime Minister Narendra Modi proposed a resolution to the 69th session of the United Nations General Assembly to establish a day to honor yoga's teachings.

Note that, prior to being elected prime minister of India, as a representative of the BJP (the conservative Bharatiya Janata Party), Modi had for almost a decade been denied a travel visa to come to the US.

Why, you might wonder? Well, international human rights organizations, like Human Rights Watch and Amnesty International, found Prime Minister Modi to be complicit in a series of violent, ethnically motivated riots that took place in February–March of 2002, in Gujarat, India, where Modi was the chief minister (akin to a state governor in the US). In these riots, masses of Hindu mobs went on a rampage and murdered hundreds of Muslim families. Neither police nor government officials intervened. The massacre is referred to by some as a pogrom because it was executed with the support of the state, and specifically targeted one ethnic group, in this case Muslims living in India. It is estimated that at least 1000, and more than likely almost 2000, Muslim mothers, families, and children were murdered by Hindu nationalist gangs; and women and children encountered other forms of brutal violence such as gang beatings and rape and torture. Ample evidence indicates that Modi – a devout Hindu nationalist – turned a blind eye and essentially condoned the targeted violence, and it was for this reason that he was for almost a decade denied a visa to attend the US.

However, once Modi was elected prime minister of India through the BJP party, President Obama and other US immigration services removed the ban on his visa and allowed him entry to the US with a diplomatic visa. And as an avid yoga practitioner himself, when Modi came to New York to attend the UN, he came with a purpose.

In his appeal to the UN members, Modi emphasized that 'yoga is an invaluable gift of India's ancient tradition', but the rhetoric of yoga being an ancient tradition lives more in our public imagination than it does in historical records. In making claims about the contribution that ancient India has made to the world, Modi also hinted at the existence of yoga as part of a timeless, Hindu culture. He also appealed to international leaders to recognize yoga as a viable solution to the global catastrophe of climate change, global terrorism, and world peace. And just prior to issuing his call for a resolution, he spoke of the threat of terrorism, and how nations like Pakistan must support India (and the West) in working toward global peace, thus hinting that terrorism is inherently connected to the threat posed by 'radical Islam'. One hundred and seventy-seven UN member nations supported Modi's motion and voted to approve the creation of his new international holiday.

Who can blame these international leaders for approving such a resolution? After all, a practice that claims to fight climate change, foster world peace, and end global terrorism while we are on the brink of ecological and nuclear disaster certainly sounds appealing.

From the point of view of racial representation, it might be deemed a good thing for International Day of Yoga to be honoring the ancient roots of yoga. But when we take a critical look, we see a more pernicious political agenda.

What are the implications of an International Day of Yoga in India? And why was the prime minister who was formerly banned from the US for crimes against humanity so intent on passing a resolution to connect yoga's 'ancient roots' to South Asia or India?

With every day that Prime Minister Modi has held his position as prime minister of India since 2014, India has been racing toward waging a genocidal attack on Muslims and other marginalized groups living in the South Asian region. Modi uses the rhetoric of decolonization to advance a political agenda of hate against religious and social minorities.

Prime Minister Modi is racialized as Brown, or South Asian. He is a person of formerly colonized ancestors. He is a South Asian who is reclaiming yoga from the Western world's culturally dominant grip on the tradition. Yet, he is also using yoga to advance an agenda of religious and ethnic nationalism.

The majority of people who use the hashtags #InternationalDayOfYoga,

#YogaDay and #InternationalYogaDay or who lead public offerings around the globe on June 21 every year are presumably well intentioned. I would also presume, however, that they are quite unaware of the ways that Prime Minister Modi is colluding with Hindu vigilante mobs – all of whom practice yoga on a daily basis – to enact genocide against Muslims living in India.

The pervasive power of *omwashing* and *orientalism* spreads even to the most appropriated forms of Western yoga. Many such yogis fail to recognize how yoga is being adapted and co-opted to legitimize ethnonationalism and state violence. The introduction of yoga programs in prisons and in the political sectors of the Indian government and United Nations programming might seem to be positive forces in the world, but I invite us as yoga teachers not to be fooled by the optics of representation – and instead consider the ethical deployment of these practices.

TOWARD A LIBERATORY YOGA

Most of the focus addressing the colonization of yoga tends to emphasize the 'whitewashing' of yoga, but I believe we can go much deeper in addressing the layers of yoga's colonization. By only thinking about how harm occurs through the representation and cultural appropriation of yoga, we miss out on addressing the ways yoga is co-opted by governments and authoritarian leaders to distract from their projects of state violence, ongoing occupation, and systems of institutionalized social hierarchy and make themselves look peaceful. We will fail at decolonizing yoga if we refuse to address these structures.

In May and June of 2021, in light of the more recent atrocities launched by the state of Israel on the people living in the occupied Palestinian territories, a few comrades and I used International Yoga Day to call on yogis to 'reimagine what spiritual and political solidarity with Palestinians, Kashmiris and all oppressed people can look like within the embodiment of one's yoga practice'. In a public solidarity statement, we repurposed the holiday to call for the abolition of colonial and state violence and move toward solidarity with the people of Palestine – and other marginalized people.[7]

While the statement received tremendous appreciation and support from yogis who already have a sharp and critical analysis of Zionism as a form of settler colonial violence, I was also deeply disappointed by the absence of support from prominent yoga teachers whose leadership in yoga spaces has been popularized by them calling out and addressing the violence of white supremacy of yoga spaces. Once it came down to them supporting and signing their name in opposition to Israeli apartheid and in support of Palestinian people, their voices were mute. This is the absence of critical thinking that I think pervades yoga spaces.

In order for yoga to be oriented toward a liberatory, futuristic vision, I believe it must be couched in a politics of *abolitionism* and *international solidarity* – and a framework of liberation theology. This would create the conditions for solidarity with Palestinians, Kashmiris, Dalits, Muslims, and all oppressed people.

13 —

ANTI-RACIST PEDAGOGY AS AN ACT OF LOVE

Simran Uppal

In our experience, while yoga teachers are becoming more aware of issues of race and justice and how they have shaped and continue to shape the practice of yoga, far fewer teachers are sure how to integrate their learning into their own work. For this chapter, Simran brings us a radically anti-racist pedagogy that is achievable as a yoga teacher. Simran makes the argument that we should experience pedagogy as an act of love, serving students while remaining deeply rooted in your needs as a teacher and as a person.

Like Sheena, Simran critiques the appropriation of representation politics by corporate equality and diversity initiatives, but this is a more practical chapter that moves beyond theory as well as beyond the tick-box exercises and performative white guilt of many courses in racial 'awareness'.

It includes a series of enquiries to help the reader move from simple analyses of structural problems to practices for personal and professional development that lead to real change. This approach: of incremental reflection, of holding space for both grief and joy, of offering dignity and uplifting others, and of putting our deepest experiences to work in fuelling change is, we believe, much more relevant to yoga teaching today.

Good anti-racist pedagogy can be many things, but it is always critical, rooted in care, solidarity, and co-creation. This chapter argues for and explores these four principles, and tries to resource you – through illustration, case study, citation, and questions – in using them to interrogate, (re)orient, or build your practice.

Maybe my first, and I think my most important mentor, Robert Lawrance, told me – showed me – as a teenager that teaching is about giving the students in the room what they need, not teaching what you want to teach. Use these four principles to equip you to find out your students' needs, and try to meet them.

At the heart of this work is, fundamentally, love. We do these things because we care, and because we want to be there for each other. Pedagogy is a very particular way of moving in love, and it does not work for everyone, or for every instance; engaging in this work is a commitment to try to move in love in your treatment of all your students, many of whom will disappoint and hurt you. Be sure that you are not harmed – in the sense of anything more substantial than a passing hurt – and be firm with your boundaries.

This is doubly true outside of formal education spaces. I recently confronted a racist, by gently calling them in to change only to have it spat back in my face. Not everyone is ready, and sometimes the correct response – for everyone involved – is to shove someone into a wall, and call them precisely those things that few publishers would give the nod to.

So, most importantly, how can the essays in this chapter and this book, and your ongoing reflective process as an educator, help you locate *your* needs, as an educator and as a person, and support the process of trying to meet them? What sort of relationships do you need? What resources are available to you, what are not, and what needs to change – in your surroundings, in yourself, and in the world – for those needs to be met?

And – maybe, in fact, very most importantly – how do you feel about that? There is a grief, of needs not having been met, of needs not currently being met, of the needs that might not or never will be met, at the heart of anti-racist education work. This grief is one of the many things at the heart of all work for liberation, for me and for a lot of people, I think. My therapist says that I speak about grief as something very liquid in my body, and he describes sadness as close to something that can unblock blockages in the bodymind. It is not for me to tell you how to meet your grief or sadnesses, and it is not for this chapter to offer ideas for how you might continue in that process.

It is for me to say this, though: this work we are talking about is constituted of turning our faces, our gaze, the focus of our individual and community attention, on violence of the worst order. This is not about trauma porn – about looking at what is terrible and feeling release or absolution from our guilt at doing nothing, or guilt invested in your whiteness or other positionality. This is about coming together to try to see what is happening in the world, in our communities, in each other and in ourselves, so we can live honestly and well, and so we can strategically, sustainably, and safely resource each other to survive, thrive, and build power for taking collective action.

So, check for that grief. Check for what is on the line for you when taking part in this work – in yourself, in your place in the world, and in the sort of life that you will or will no longer be happy living. Educators have a special responsibility to at least be aware of as many of the dark corners of the world and of themselves as possible, and this may not be a safe, sustainable, or strategically effective use of the energies that you have. Look frankly at the resourcing, care, supervision, mentoring, and other support that you have, for your work, yourself, and your health, and make a decision. Under-resourced, under-supervised educators, who are not able to face up in honest enough ways to themselves and the world around them, do not have a special place in hell. We do not believe in retributive hells here; we believe in transformative justice. What's clear, though, is that those educators create a hell in our collective here and now, for themselves and those who place themselves, vulnerably, in their care.

FIRST REFLECTIONS

1. This is about strategy. It is about theories of change, and it is about creating communities that can dream answers and fight for them, sustainably. What do you need to locate and carry out a good role for you?
2. This is about needs. What are yours – as a person, and as an educator? What are the needs of each of your individual students, as people, and as political agents?
3. This is about agency. Building power to exercise change happens by facilitating and resourcing individuals to stand in their agency – as much through mutual aid, basic security, and care work as through conversation and strategy. How do your students relate to their agency in your teaching spaces? How are you participating in that?
4. This is about care. What care is needed for the political education work you want to do – for yourself, and for participants? Who does that care work, and who doesn't have (sufficient) access to it?

ESTABLISHING A RADICAL APPROACH

We need a radical, critical approach. This is about critical pedagogy, not about equality, diversity, and inclusion trainings. We'll start with two citations, one from Paulo Freire, and one from Emma Dabiri. Paulo Freire, who died in 1997, established critical pedagogy as an approach to education, and as a first Brazilian, then soon global, movement for political change:

> But almost always, during the initial stage of the struggle, the oppressed, instead of striving for liberation, tend themselves to become oppressors, or 'sub-oppressors'. The very structure of their thought has been conditioned by the contradictions of the concrete, existential situation by which they were shaped. Their ideal is to be humans; but for them, to be humans is to be oppressors.[1]

bell hooks, who builds on Freire's work to form what she calls 'engaged pedagogy' – perhaps a whisper of Thich Nhat Hanh's Engaged Buddhism, of which she was a great admirer and practitioner – names her book on the subject *Teaching to Transgress: Education as a Practice of Freedom* (1994).[2] Emma Dabiri is a sociologist, and among many other things, the author of *What White People Can Do Next: From Allyship to Coalition* (2021).[3] She describes this as a Trojan Horse: a sort of bait-and-switch, with a title in line with the various liberal, vigourless anti-racist guides for white people, but content in line with the Black radical tradition and anti-imperial Marxisms. 'It's not just about making white people nicer through cajoling, begging, demanding, imploring, training – it's actually about challenging racial taxonomy and concepts such as whiteness.'[4]

But almost always, during the initial stage of the struggle, the oppressed, instead of striving for liberation, tend themselves to become oppressors, or 'sub-oppressors'. The very structure of their thought has been conditioned by the contradictions of the concrete, existential situation by which they were shaped. Their ideal is to be humans; but for them, to be humans is to be oppressors.[5]

In 2019, UK Black Pride and Stonewall launched a campaign, 'Proudly Pro-You', in partnership with Nyx Cosmetics, a subsidiary of L'Oréal. The campaign itself seemed positive, and more substantial than many similar partnerships: as well as an advertising campaign with five emerging queer creatives of colour, the campaign announced a listening campaign, to support their intentions of distributing grants to community organizations supporting queer people of colour in the UK. The advertising campaign beautifully celebrated and platformed the work of a diverse set of five young, talented queer people of colour. I often think how much suffering I would have avoided if posters of people like me had been up on the billboards on the way to school, and it always warms my heart to see *apne*, my own people, doing well. Well-distributed grants (I've struggled to find further details, but am happy to take it on faith) are also a cause for celebration; post-austerity Britain is a place where few community organizations are flush with funding.

This is a success of diversity, of inclusion, and – in the distribution of funding – likely supportive of equality. Before I move to criticism, though, I think it is essential to recognize the pressure to fall into black-and-white thinking. You may wish to take a moment of somatic awareness or other contemplation as I begin to discuss the ways in which the campaign was a failure, and/or actively harmful. How easy is it to hold polarities, to hold seeming opposites? Why the desire to reconcile everything into one or the other? Does it become more possible to hold both, if we give our grief and anger full space, too?

It is finally worth noting that the approach to anti-racism found most widely in the yoga and wellness sectors today, and more widely – one of EDI,[i] or some version of that – emerges not from grassroots community organizing radical, transformative social change work, or even from the work of a well-meaning sociologist. It comes from corporate boardrooms, liberal non-profits restricted by the demands of their funders, and a scattering of politically disengaged academics working with minimal awareness of the rich histories of political education and critical pedagogy present in the UK and globally.

L'Oréal, the company behind Nyx, is the biggest cosmetics company in the world by revenue. In 2008, the BDS movement – Boycott, Divestment, Sanctions, the most globally influential voice of Palestinian civil society, a campaign opposed to Israeli settler colonialism and apartheid – added L'Oréal to their boycott list. The depth of L'Oréal's business and other relations with Israel is extraordinary: they continue to operate a factory out of an ethnically cleansed, apartheid-enforced village in Lower Galilee, where Palestinians are not allowed to buy, rent, or live in any part of the town. L'Oréal also manufactures and exports Dead Sea cosmetics products from the occupied West Bank; Israel prevents Palestinian access to the lake and its resources, while benefiting financially and in image from tourism and exports, just like those made by L'Oréal. Even this is the tip of the iceberg; in 2014, L'Oréal sent toiletry care packages to women in the Israeli military, while Palestinians in Gaza were

---

i   Equity, diversity, and inclusion (EDI) programmes as indicative of invariably superficial corporate attempts at anti-racist trainings.

deprived of access to electricity and clean water by those very same soldiers. It is impossible to get clear numbers on what percentage of people in Gaza have direct access to clean water. There are obviously just as many queers in Gaza as there are anywhere else. I am unsure how you square the circle when a transnational corporation (nearly 30 billion euros turnover last year) says they are 'proudly for you', given this context.

L'Oréal is also the same company that fired Munroe Bergdorf in 2017. Bergdorf is a prominent anti-racist advocate and model, a biracial Black British trans woman, who had tweeted strong words about white complicity in violence, and the nature of white supremacy. An online harassment campaign, accusing her of racism against white people, followed, after which point she was fired by L'Oréal, and continued to experience online abuse.

Stonewall is a liberally positioned, registered charity focused on advocacy for inclusion, and campaigns for legal reform. UK Black Pride are the organizers of an extraordinary yearly celebration, founded to create a radical, anti-racist space, and are supportive of but not extensively involved in political campaigning and community organizing. They have a (deservedly) prominent role in the British queer-of-colour world, as the best-known organization that represents our very varied communities.

In earlier drafts of this essay, I worked through this case study. I considered just formulating the key questions that need to be asked here – and I will – but it's important to know that these can only be illustrative. What are the questions *you* need to ask here? *Why?* What are the questions that the anti-racist 'educators' you might follow on Instagram would – or rather, would *not* ask – and, again, *why?*

What does it mean to fight for status, power, or wealth, in a system where each of those exists not just alongside the oppression of others, but dependent specifically on the *extraction* of those things from others? Do we want to climb up higher on a ladder built out of the bones of our ancestors, maintained by the snatching of bones out of the flesh of our siblings in every moment, or do we want to dismantle the ladder? How can we build the collective power to confront and stop those who are ripping the bones out from under the skin?

Who are the people in the past who have built movements that have been able to do this, to put up the fight, and to do the good work? I think of Black Marxists in the USA and across the world, community organizers in Southall, grassroots trade unionists organizing precarious workers today, anti-caste feminist worker collectives in India, anti-imperialist revolutionaries in Burkina Faso, liberation theology communities of poets and farmers in Nicaragua. There are so many huge and diverse histories of extraordinary work, and many more that have gone unarchived or erased, all underpinned by the conviction that deeper and profound change is possible, or at least worth fighting for. Reading Paulo Freire is a good place to start.

KEY PRINCIPLES OF CRITICAL PEDAGOGY IN YOGA/CONTEMPLATIVE SPACES

1. Who has the answers? Who is creating the questions? What are the horizons of possibility, the limits to what can be imagined, on the questions that are being asked?
2. What tools have given you liberating moments of insight? What was the effect, and why did each tool have that effect on you in that moment?
3. What skills do you have already that you could apply to this purpose? Think about humour, storytelling, somatic tools, think about exploring feelings and sensations in the body, listening to the smallest flickers of hesitation, anger. Think about tools from your other fields of practice – therapeutic, arts practice, other forms of education, working with young people, raising young people, raising yourself, teaching experiential anatomy, comparing translations of the same spiritual text to find the ideological slants, structuring rest into a yoga class when you know your students don't feel confident enough in their agency to rest themselves.
4. What are the questions your students need to be asking? What are the questions they are afraid to ask, and why? What are the questions they do not even know exist?

WHAT IS SOLIDARITY?

Workers of the world, unite![6]

Solidarity encompasses types of knowing, types of feeling, and types of action. It stems from the knowledge that the freedom and wellbeing of each of us is inseparable from the freedom and wellbeing of all others; the knowledge that our liberation is a shared one. It is achieved by caring with, caring alongside, caring *as*, not caring *for* – it is liberatory, collective, co-creative, and not paternalistic. And action that is born from these or that produces these is action from and in order to build agency, particularly in those places where agency is most diminished and harm is most present.

REFLECTIONS ON SOLIDARITY

The following exercises invite direct reflection on the presence of oppression and organized forms of harm and exploitation in your life. Choose your moment well. Remember that vulnerability describes a state where you know you are resourced to recover even if the worst should happen; anything else is recklessness at best, or perhaps a destructive drive at worst.

1. If you are white, think of the ways that whiteness diminishes your ability to live well. This may be in the way it meets and reinforces other oppressions: of class, of gender, of disability, of queerness. This may be in the way it seeps into your life: how is your soul not able to be light, as is its birth right, because of the weight of harm working in and through the world you live in, and even – perhaps – through you and your ancestors?

2. Whiteness was created to bolster the extraction of resources from people of colour, in order to support the ever-growing stolen wealth of the wealthiest. Where do you stand in relation to this, as a person of colour?

3. Whiteness was created, operates by, and recreates itself, by exerting control, violence, and harm through huge systems that organize how money moves through the world, how humans move or do not move past lines drawn in soil, ocean, or barbed wire, what we do or do not have access to, and how we perceive ourselves and each other. Where do you stand in relation to this, whoever you are?

Thomas Sankara, the first president of Burkina Faso and leader of one of the most successful anti-imperialist, Marxist governments ever seen, once wrote:

I speak on behalf of all those who seek in vain for a forum in the world where they can be heard. Yes, I wish to speak for all those – the forgotten – because I am a man and nothing that is human is alien to me.[7]

Anti-racist pedagogy needs to take this at its heart; we are not trying to tax-onomize ourselves further, or alienate ourselves from each other further, or alienate ourselves from ourselves even further. We are looking directly at the systems of taxonomy (whiteness and all that comes with it), oppression, and alienation, and finding ways to participate in the fight against them.

If you find yourself, as a non-South Asian yoga teacher, asking whether you should be teaching yoga, you will find so many resources through this text. My first thought is always that we need to severely problematize the ideas of yoga's pure, Indian-read-Hindu mythic history, and think more about the evidence for its transnational formations. This is about the influence of Hindutva, of the Hindu ethnonationalist, murderous, far-right fascist central government and its projects in the worlds of academia and global soft power work, as Sheena Sood discusses so well.

But it goes beyond this: why should this question be so centred? What benefits can you bring through teaching, to people of colour as much as to anyone else? What harm is caused to Muslim, low-caste, and other non-hegemonic yoga teachers and practitioners, by the idea that yoga is only by and for high-caste Hindus and those who bow to their authority? In fact – why is the focus on whether or not you should teach yoga, and not on where else in life you can build a sustainable and meaningful practice of solidarity? If you are a full-time yoga teacher on a low income, dealing with precarious working conditions, scrabbling to get by, at constant risk of harm – maybe the question is: how can I move in solidarity with other members of this new working class? You will find out quickly that most of the precarious workers in our new economy – Uber drivers, cleaners, couriers, even foster care workers – are people of colour, too. Fighting for your rights, as a worker, means standing in solidarity with some of the most exploited groups of people of colour in this country, and worldwide.

CARE AND CO-CREATION

Rest isn't something we can force, or 'make' happen. Rest is a spontaneous experience. We can only cultivate the conditions for it to arise within.

Harriet McAtee[8]

Questions on education rooted in care

1. How could you factor rest into your session structure?
2. Is there any way to imagine anti-racist education as a restful experience?

3. Is your current anti-racist pedagogy practice sustainable? What patterns of action and rest are predominant in the social change work you do, and how do you feel about them?
4. How do you relate to *pleasure* in your work, and how might its absence make your work unsustainable?
5. What ways have you successfully met or worked with the care needs of a participant? What ways have you failed to do so? Which participants do you find attending your sessions, which ones do not, and why?

Radical education can only happen well in spaces in which we feel safe, and those in which we are well resourced and looked after, as full persons. Considering the elements of *care work* that are present in your teaching is a useful way to working towards that, and a way to make this work sustainable, for you and for your students. The politics and practice of care are inseparable from the politics of and practice towards accessibility, particularly within matrices of gender and disability. This is clearest through illustration.

Incomplete checklist for care and accessibility in anti-racist pedagogy

- Sufficiently frequent, sufficiently long rest breaks.
- Sufficient processes for making sure you know how much rest students are likely to need.
- Integration of rest and/or self-care practices into or around more challenging or potentially triggering work.
- Content notes or trigger warnings, placed or timed to give sufficient warning; class outlines prior to sessions, particularly when potentially challenging elements are included.
- Orientation towards 'opt-in' rather than 'opt-out', wherever possible.
- Maximum physical and/or digital access: hybrid sessions to enable participation from shielding students, gender-neutral toilet facilities, properly installed ramps and handrails, public transport and/or taxi funding, food, water, and quiet spaces, British Sign Language (BSL) interpretation and/or live captioning, large-print and/or audio-recorded textual materials...
- Crèche spaces; timings around the school day and school year; flexibility in longer courses, for participation from those with diverse and/or complex long-term carer responsibilities.

- Tiered pricing; solidarity/bursary funds; collaboration with mutual aid and/or community food provision services.
- Orientation towards co-creation, collaboration, and facilitation.

The final item on this incomplete checklist is perhaps the most important. Care is a relational behaviour; accessibility is a relational right – that is, care is something that happens in interpersonal relationships, and accessibility is rooted in the relationship between each individual and a wider group. Finding appropriate ways of relating to each other is at the core of doing this work well; it's at the core of doing, I would say, with Theo Wildcroft, any form of yoga teaching or teaching well.

Questions for co-creative teaching

1. What is the purpose of planning a session? What benefit is there in planning less, or more? When is a plan a support, and when is it a shield?
2. What is on the line for you in not presenting yourself as an authority?
3. When was the last time you picked a fight with someone telling you what to do? What can you do today to reconnect to that energy? How could you connect to that energy in a session?
4. What planning tools can you use to enable greater flexibility? Can you sketch the session in a non-linear way? Could you imagine key ideas as elements in chords, chord progressions, flavours in a complex dish, colours in an impressionist painting, rather than paragraphs? What other directions, flavours, colours, notes, might go well?

There are brilliant essays in this collection on this very topic, but for here, we could simply highlight three parts: on listening, respecting, and even facilitating each other's agency, and working interactively – subversively – with the authority or power that you hold in a space as a teacher, respected figure, or facilitator. This is how we co-create the protocols needed in each space; this is how we move towards safety and care, by working gently and slowly to put individual and collective agency back at the centre of our work.

This is, I think, at the heart of experiencing pedagogy as a form of love. There is a shared intimacy and honesty in this sort of space; a spaciousness that enables closeness as and when it is right for us. It is alright, I think, to be afraid of these spaces, and I grieve for all those who are too afraid to give this a try – to bring whatever protectors they have inside them home.

On the other side of this grief and its siblings is the most extraordinary pleasure, and plenty of suffering. Pleasure like climbing the wall of a rock-climbing gym and reaching a hold only with the cheers and shouted advice of your friends, and suffering like slipping off and grazing all down your shins, but knowing – at some level – there's time and plasters enough for healing. Work that is in line with love and honesty, love as an active, bell-hooks-ian practice, as the no-fear, carry a sword at your hip devotion of my Sikh ancestors is itself a liberation. It is itself a way of meeting the there and then of freedom that we dream of here in our everyday lives, in the communities we move in or even are privileged enough to build, even before the whole battle is won.

14

BREATHING OUT LOUD

Aisha Nash

Aisha Nash became a yoga teacher after leaving a career as an award-winning pastry chef. After practising with her mum as a child, she re-discovered yoga first as a way to rehabilitate after an injury, then to help her be entirely content with exactly the person she is. When she wanted to share her yoga practice with others, she found that she didn't fit the mould of a yoga teacher that studios were looking for, and began creating safe spaces for anyone who might have similar experiences walking into a yoga studio. Aisha now teaches classes that are focused on inclusivity, diversity, and self-love, with what she calls her Anti-Diet Yoga Approach.

Once again, we wanted a more personal reflection on the theme to end this section. One of Aisha's many gifts is in personalizing the impact of racism in yoga through the intimacy of bodily experience. In this chapter, she describes the violence that is done through our racialized assumptions about what a 'healthy' body looks and feels like. Black women and femme-presenting people suffer this alienation from white 'health' and 'femininity' in so many aspects of our shared culture. But just as in our section on trauma, Aisha shows us how the intersection of yoga and race can be used in the service of either appropriative harm or reclaimed healing. This chapter describes a personal journey, unpeeling the layers of hypocrisy and violence in the wellness industry, and experiencing the grief, rage, and empowerment that results.

At the age of five, I remember learning to do a shoulder stand and put my legs into lotus.

A year later, a family member commented on the size of my thighs...at 14, a much younger cousin said I had a fat stomach...17, a boy said I was too big for him to date...18, I went to the first yoga studio to open in my area, and the teacher pointed out I breathed wrong.

I had spent my whole life, up until 18, trying desperately to suck in my belly so much that I had never taken a full inhale.

At 18, I learnt to nourish my body with deep breaths and even louder exhales.

The backbone of my life, from childhood to adulthood, was about controlling my physical body.

I learnt the most important thing I could ever do in society was to be thin – to take up less space.

At 19, I started weight lifting. I had never enjoyed anything more in my life. My days were filled with meal prepping, and ensuring I was fuelled enough to pick up and put down increasingly heavier weights.

At 21, I stopped – partially from my career choice, but mostly because I would be teased about being 'too muscular' to be a girl...even though I was already an adult woman. But you know that what the aesthetic society requires at all times is for women to look like children; small, slim, hairless (in some areas), and most of all, weak.

I remember reading a book when I was younger, about a woman going through the throes of an eating disorder; I read every book, multiple times, learning behaviours from them. I remember the quote 'Some people who are obsessed with food become gourmet chefs. Others become eating disordered.'

I decided to do the former. It was such a demanding occupation, that any form of physical activity that was for myself disappeared. I worked 16-hour days, five days a week. It was such a mentally and emotionally exhausting job, I didn't even have the capacity to exercise or focus on dieting. No wonder it only took five years for me to burn out.

I ran back to yoga to heal myself. It was the only thing that through my life had felt in any way healing. So, I poured my heart and soul into physically practising all I could.

And here starts the real journey of disordered eating and being immersed into a shallow, self-obsessed world. Filled with more hypocrisy than I'd ever come across before.

I was compared continuously to an ideal I could not attain and I took that as a personal fault. When you grow up as a woman in this image-obsessed society, you take on every person's dislike and bigotry as your own failure, and I blamed what I looked like for not getting jobs, not being given opportunities that were given to people with less training than me, and I thought I could change their opinion, if only I could look the part. If only I were skinny enough.

I did every diet, every wellness trend. I followed every lifestyle change, until eventually, this ex-chef was scared of eating in restaurants.

Restaurants were where I became an adult, where I learnt hard work, and creativity, where I honed friendships that still carry on to this day, and I adore them. I used to feel at home in restaurants; not just the kitchen, but the finely attuned theatre that is good service and plating.

The whole thing was magic for me.

It was not only me in this cycle of trying to shrink myself. I was surrounded by people thinner, whiter, and more flexible, all still trying every diet, every 'wellness' trend, in the hope that this one would be the magic bullet to give them the body and life that they desired. I didn't understand; their bodies were the ones plastered all over the walls.

They were the ideal that everyone was trying to match.

Seeing this, seeing people much thinner than me beating themselves with the same stick made me question their behaviour. They were yoga teachers – looked to by their students as paragons of health who should be leading by example, but they smoked and did lines in the bathroom. Seeing that it was not and never had been about being healthy – only about being thin – snapped me out of my desire to trade everything for thinness. I knew I had done unhealthy things, like starve myself, but I had never gone that far, and seeing it in reality showed me that thinness did not equate to health.

In the same way I would devour the latest book on dieting, I took that focus and turned it into probing the research behind this ideal that we are all held to. I wanted to know if diets worked, and along this journey I found out about intuitive eating, and about the racist reasons we have these body ideals.

And when I started to embrace my body as it is and challenged the harmful messages being promoted in yoga spaces, I got fired.

The best thing that ever happened to me, bar meeting my husband, was being fired from this toxic place.

Working at other yoga studios, I found that it was the same, but less image obsessed. Instead, the toxicity came from cultural appropriation, in the form of a weird attachment to the appearance of a spirituality which was taken out of context. Statues of Ganesh in the bathroom, Shiva above the radiator, and incense everywhere. While the aesthetics of these places were Indian-inspired, they never seemed to care about India, yoga, or even the statues that they had bought. There was an attachment to looking the part, but no follow-through or respect for the culture that was making them a lot of money.

At the same time as this, I was undergoing what is best described as an awakening; learning about the diet industry, the Eurocentric body ideals that have shaped diet culture, and (what surprised me the most) the insidious racism these ideals are based on.

If I had never stopped dieting, if I didn't have the free mental space, I never would've noticed these things.

I would've only blamed myself for the problems instead of noticing that the company culture at these places was so completely messed up.

I gradually began to learn this wasn't just happening in yoga studios. It was happening in grocery shops, in all fitness studios and spaces, and it was capitalizing on ancient wellness traditions that have existed in many places, being practised by Indigenous populations whose connection to these practices was being side-lined. Worse still, many Indigenous people would have been killed or otherwise punished for these practices during the height of colonialism.

I read *Fearing the Black Body* by Dr Sabrina Strings and it woke me up even more. I was suddenly surrounded by people who felt the same way I did. People who loved the practice, but were questioning the way it is taught and rebelling against what is deemed as 'authentic' yoga in the West. They inspired me and taught me so much, and I love that I get to call them my friends and teachers. We'd get together once a month (in those magical pre-pandemic days) and hug it out. We'd hold space for how much this continued colonization of our heritage hurt. We'd be honest for the first time about how soul-sucking it is to fit into a mould that does not fit, because it was never made to fit us – only to stifle and silence us, and profit from our pain.

I learnt about the inherent anti-Blackness that was involved in creating the body ideals of today. The way thinkers from the so-called 'Enlightenment' period were not very enlightened at all. The way that they kidnapped, stole, pillaged, and degraded not only ideas but people, and treated them in ways so horrific I cannot write them down for fear you and I both will not recover from the tears we'll shed. For those slightly curious, I recommend you start by simply Googling the word 'drapetomania'.

I learnt that when the transatlantic slave trade ended, that was not the end of people being enslaved. That when more labourers were required, hundreds and thousands of Indians were tricked into becoming indentured servants. Slavery never really ended, the name was simply changed, and that change in language mirrors what goes on now. It's mirrored in the self-care rhetoric taught to us through social media. No longer is a bath something that you do to clean your body; now it is an action of 'self-care' and made a capitalist thing by adverts reminding you of needing a 12-step skincare routine and your bath bomb. Now your lunch break is not a human decency; it's a treat to take a break away from your desk. Now simply movement, something inherent to all animals on this earth, is being sold back to you as 'somatics'. Now humans have to have multiple jobs to simply earn the minimum they require to afford a roof over their head, and it's praised as 'hustling' or 'grinding', and this culture has invaded yoga spaces.

Ask any yoga teacher how many studios they have to teach at, how often they have to beg for new classes, what their other jobs are, or how many companies have only paid them in 'exposure'.

(I've checked with my bank – this is not a recognized currency for paying bills with.)

Everything has been rebranded to make it a viable product, including the wellness industry. We can't even eat fruit now without the decision being made much more complicated and costly.

This rebranding strategy that is part white supremacy, part capitalism, has caused yoga to become a shell of what it was, and also requires its yoga teachers to appear as a vapid shell of toxic positivity.

I have found while working in this career that any time I tried to step away from that stereotype, there was the stick of losing a class, thus ensuring you stay silent so you can carry on paying rent. Even when they seemed to be in support of intersectional equity, they were often only paying lip service to the words a diversity, equality, and inclusion (DEI) consultant had told them, never implementing real change.

The entire yoga industry – from the ashrams in India to the Yoga Alliance schools in the UK – desperately need to pledge their allegiance to becoming actively anti-racist. There needs to be a serious look at how anti-Black the wellness industry is within its actions and the things it sells to us.

Only by embracing an anti-racist stance could there be any change at all, and it needs to be a systemic, top-down, and bottom-up change. It's not enough to make it an option; it needs to be mandatory for hiring professionals, and the stance needs to be internalized by all those in leadership positions.

Fifteen per cent of the UK's population is encased in the grossly exclusionary phrase 'BAME' – Black and minority ethnic. If you are white and reading this, think about that – the global *majority* of the world are referred to by this acronym, or BIPOC (Black and Indigenous people of colour). In both of these, white people are centred – everyone who is not white is grouped together, regardless of their distinguishable ethnicities, cultures, or religions. For a company to only talk about supporting or addressing the needs of BAME or

BIPOC can be functionally meaningless unless they care enough to find out about the individuals that will be affected by such policies.

This shows up every time a yoga studio wants to diversify its portfolio of teachers. They'll hire one or two Black or brown people, and not look further into the company and industry culture that created a space that mostly only white people feel safe to be as teachers or students. This creates a further culture of harm for racially minoritized people (a term coined by sociologist Dr Yasmin Gunaratnum) and once again ensures fewer non-white teachers in such places and spaces.

These ideas of human beings that are not white, yet having their life revolve around the ideals that white European men have created, are at the core of what we call diet culture. These institutions that we want to work at, that we study at, that we live surrounded by are owned by old rich white men, and that means that if the global majority aren't conforming to such twisted ideals, they are oppressed, and even when they try their best to conform, they are held back.

This rhetoric that everything that is white is more important than anything living and breathing is shown in the bills being passed in the UK parliament; laws that protect statues and give longer sentences to protestors and those who harm statues than those who rape and murder human beings.

These harmful ideologies of whiteness, nationalism, and diet culture are clung to so fervently and tightly that we even have the phrase 'the obesity paradox' to explain away the fact that scientific research has shown that being obese is medically insignificant, and in fact it is the so-called 'underweight' category that has the highest mortality rate and worse health outcomes overall.

How can we claim a home and a safe place in our bodies, when they are deemed less important than statues of slave masters?

How can we begin to live a life feeling grateful for our bodies, when whole body types and skin colours are vilified for existing?

Politics affects us all, and will continue to do so, because on a larger scale, it allows those who are privileged to keep their privilege, without being aware of their privilege. It also keeps the rest of us in a place of hustling and grinding to simply keep a roof over our heads.

Think about the average yoga studio attendee... What can you see in your mind? What is their body type? Their skin colour, their socioeconomic status...?

Based on my experience, I highly doubt that you are imagining a person from a marginalized background, living in anything other than a thin/able body, or from a lower socioeconomic status...

... And that's the problem.

MONEY AND POWER

15 __

YOGA MEANS UNION

Laura Hancock

Laura Hancock is the co-creator of the Yoga Teachers Union (a branch of the IWGB), the first trade union for yoga teachers in the UK. After a number of years working in the charity sector, she qualified as a yoga teacher in 2012, followed shortly by Ayurvedic massage therapy in 2013. One of Laura's great passions is how care and wellbeing are valued, supported, and integrated into our society, how we interrelate as a community, and how we each move through the world. In 2019 she co-founded the Oxford Wellbeing Cooperative – a diverse collective of practitioners who are working towards sustainable and accessible wellbeing support to the Oxford community. Forming the Yoga Teachers Union was the logical conclusion of turning that instinct for sustainability issues back on the profession itself.

When we approached Laura to write this piece, we knew the result would be uncompromising. Laura and her union colleagues were supporting members with cases of burnout, precarity, bullying, and sexual harassment. This chapter is, we believe, a much-needed and clearly demonstrated reframing of yoga teachers as workers in a gig economy, wrestling with the vagaries of late-stage capitalism. Yoga teaching for many is a spiritual practice in itself, and a caring profession by choice and design. But it is also a vulnerable, stressful profession for many.

In this piece, Laura demonstrates how, when we only see yoga teaching as an act of service and altruism, we provide cover for unfair pay and even illegal conditions, justified in the name of 'community' and 'service'. In truth, the precarity of most yoga teaching is a heavy burden, complicated by the societal undervaluing of all caring professions. She argues that collective action and legal redress are the only way for yoga teachers to gain the recognition and rights that we deserve.

In October 2020 the Yoga Teachers' Branch of the IWGB had its inaugural meeting and officially became the first yoga teachers trade union (YTU) in the UK, and I was elected founding chair. Not only was this the first time that yoga teachers had organized in this way, it also established yoga as an industry, and one that is populated by workers who are vulnerable enough to need a union. As Sarah Jaffe states in her explanation of class composition, yoga teachers had begun to consider their relationship to power within the industry, and to identify themselves as workers.

The formation of the union captured the attention of media outlets across the world, and began to challenge public misconceptions of yoga, bringing to light the fact that the yoga industry, just like every other unregulated industry, is exploitative. We, as Davy states in the next chapter, are not in a bubble. We are not special. We are workers, just like everyone else.

There's no succinct or obvious route into the vast and complex topic of capitalism, the gig economy, and workers' rights, but a trade union lens focuses on power and vulnerability to exploitation. With that focus there are some key issues that have repeatedly emerged, and common beliefs that form distinct barriers to yoga teachers organizing for better working conditions. They are:

1. Yoga teaching is a spiritual practice. This implies that seeking remuneration for our teaching is unspiritual.
2. Yoga teachers are carers and working from a place of love. This implies that seeking remuneration for our teaching is uncaring and not loving.
3. Yoga teachers choose to be self-employed. This implies that joining a union would remove our freedom and autonomy.

In order to address the topic of capitalism, workers' rights, and the gig economy it is imperative that we take a closer look at these three statements. This is an opportunity to recalibrate how we identify ourselves. We are workers trying to survive within a highly competitive, hyper-individualistic, precarious, and exploitative capitalist society.

For clarity's sake, the definition of capitalism is, as per the Oxford Dictionary, 'An economic and political system in which a country's trade and industry are controlled by private owners for profit, rather than by the state.'[1] Some sources estimate that the current worth of the yoga industry is $84 billion USD globally.[i] Yet yoga teachers are struggling to get by. When surveying yoga teachers across the UK in 2019 about working conditions the most striking findings were that:[2]

- 76 per cent said that they didn't have a contract, and of those that did the majority stated that they felt the contracts were in the venue's favour and they felt little to no protection
- over 60 per cent stated that they were struggling to earn a sustainable living.

A further study in July 2020 evidenced significant loss of income due to Covid, further heightening levels of precarity.[3] This study also found that on average yoga teachers work an additional two hours for every hour they teach. Yoga teachers have every reason to organize and to address the power imbalances within the industry.

YOGA TEACHING IS SEEN AS A SPIRITUAL PRACTICE. THIS IMPLIES THAT SEEKING REMUNERATION FOR OUR TEACHING IS UNSPIRITUAL.

Donna Farhi explores this sensitive and often polarizing topic in the chapter 'The Ethics of Money' in her 2006 book, *Teaching Yoga*. She emphasizes the relationship between student and teacher and discusses the importance of accepting that in Western culture and society, value and worth are measured by financial exchange. She argues that to deny this reality, at the expense of the wellbeing and livelihood of the teacher, is more revealing of those who pose the question, than the teachers themselves:

> When we do business in a way which everyone prospers and is nourished and rewarded, it is one of the highest ways of putting our spirituality to the test. The argument that a teacher asking for a fair exchange for services is not being spiritual is often a projection by the accuser, who is unwilling to be fair and equitable in his own dealings and is looking for justification for his own greed.[4]

---

i   See 'What "everyone" knows about yoga' in the Introduction for discussion of this and other similar statistics.

In applying this to the relationship between venue owner/manager and teacher, the same pattern emerges. Members of the union repeatedly raise concerns about bullying, silencing, and unfair employment practices being masked behind spiritual terminology and narratives. It is worth noting that this type of behaviour occurs across the whole spectrum of workplaces, and has been predominantly reported from independent, community-focused studios. The belief that exploitation is limited to big corporations isn't consistent with my experience as chair and case worker of the union.

I can draw from my own personal experience to demonstrate this. When seeking remuneration for six weeks' worth of teaching at a local, independent studio phrases such as 'you need to look at your money trauma' and 'you should be teaching from love, not fear' were used to detract from my very reasonable demands for basic payment terms. I remember clearly how vulnerable I felt in that situation. My rent and utilities bills were overdue and what I thought was going to be a straightforward professional negotiation to settle unpaid work and any miscommunications became a personal attack on my integrity as a teacher and my apparent unresolved trauma. I needed the manager to pay me for the work that I'd done, but I had no leverage or standing. I felt a deep sense of shame and humiliation in having to beg for money in the middle of a bustling cafe. It was only with the encouragement of a non-yoga, business-minded friend that I had the confidence to persevere and eventually get paid what I was owed. I was 'let go' almost immediately afterwards for not having the 'yoga' and 'community' spirit that was expected of teachers in the venue. This experience was one of my motivations for getting so heavily involved with the union.

I am not alone in this experience. Time and time again I hear of similar behavioural patterns within the venue/teacher dynamic. I would argue that the denial of capitalism in the world of yoga is creating an accountability vacuum that risks encouraging and enabling abusive dynamics and behaviour. Such behaviour may start with financial and contractual issues, but can quickly escalate to far more destructive and violent abuses.

After discussing industry employment issues and vulnerabilities with a pro-bono employment law barrister he emailed me with this follow-up:

> I was thinking some more about what you said about the interface between the spiritual and mundane regulation. I was reminded of the strict practical rules set out by Dogen, so that the Japanese monks could live and flourish side-by-side without falling out with each other. In an ideal world we wouldn't need rules; but we are not ideal.[5]

YOGA TEACHERS ARE CARERS AND WORKING FROM A PLACE OF LOVE. THIS IMPLIES THAT SEEKING REMUNERATION FOR OUR TEACHING IS UNCARING AND NOT LOVING.

In one of my first one-to-one yoga classes I was teaching a male student in a garden shed. I was anxious and keen to impress, struggling quite heavily with this relatively new experience of self-employment, and still grappling with the recognition that this was work, for which I should get paid. Nerves aside, I felt the class had gone quite well and experienced a rush of relief as we rolled up the mats and discussed potential future bookings. Then we got to the payment. The student, who was older, stronger, and significantly more financially stable than me, placed a £20 note in my hand, and just as I was about to accept, he withdrew the note and asked me, 'How does it feel to get paid for something that should be offered from the heart?' To this day, over ten years later, I can still feel the heat in my face and chest as I tried to explain the training I'd had and the skill and experience required to do this work, essentially justifying my right to be paid. I remember becoming acutely aware of the fact that I was alone, in a shed, with a man exerting power over me.

When I shared this story many years later at a panel talk with Sarah Jaffe and fellow trade unionists of the IWGB there was a resounding cry of empathic anger. This is a particular challenge that so many workers in caring professions and industries face, and one in which gender imbalances cannot be ignored. As Jaffe describes:

> The working class is not a stable entity or a fixed category. It is, rather, a thing that changes as conditions change, as capitalism changes and produces new work ethics to match its demands. The process we call 'class composition' occurs as the workers whose labor and lives have been organised by capitalism begin to understand themselves as a class and to act accordingly in their collective interests. We can see the process happening now, as workers who might have assumed themselves middle-class start to understand that their relationship to power means they're still workers.[6]

Yoga teachers are not only faced with the challenge of realizing that we are workers within our own industry; as a predominantly woman/non-binary workforce we are also faced with the challenge of being valued within the highly patriarchal trade union, and wider workers' rights movement itself. We simply can't unionize effectively without developing a better understanding of our role and worth as carers, who are often women and non-binary workers, and how these facets of our work exacerbate our vulnerability to exploitation.

Diemut Bubeck, the author of *Care, Gender and Justice* (1995), defines care as 'an activity or practice aimed at the meeting of needs in others, whilst involving an investment of the carers' time and energy'.[7] Through surveying yoga teachers in the UK the union has established that we are, on average, working an additional two hours for every hour we are paid for, and are also often struggling to earn a sustainable living.[8] Qualitative data from the same survey also revealed the impact this was having on mental and physical health. Numerous teachers expressed deep concerns about burnout, exhaustion, and ill health as a direct result of the strains of extensive travel and gruelling schedules. Extensive emotional labour and a sense of responsibility and duty of care of students beyond the mat were also prevalent.

In *Anarchafeminism* (2022), Chiara Bottici discusses the concept of 'super-exploitation',[9] first coined by Maria Miles:[10]

> Perceiving women's labour as simply the necessary calling of their 'womanhood' instead of seeing it as the actual work it is, is pivotal to keeping the division between 'waged labor' subject to exploitation, and 'unwaged labor', subject to what she called 'super-exploitation'. This form of gendered exploitation is 'super' because, whereas the exploitation of waged labor takes place through the extraction of surplus value, the exploitation of women's domestic labor takes place via denying their work the very status of work.[11]

Whilst this statement is referring to women's labour in the home, the explicit reference to challenging the right to remuneration for work that comes 'from the heart' demonstrates its relevance to our profession, and for the gig economy and trade union landscape within which we are trying to organize.

YOGA TEACHERS CHOOSE TO BE SELF-EMPLOYED. THIS IMPLIES THAT JOINING A UNION WOULD REMOVE OUR FREEDOM AND AUTONOMY.

The results of the 2019 survey showed that approximately 60 per cent of yoga teachers were in support of the formation of a union. Of the 35 per cent who were undecided, the main deterrent was uncertainty around how we could unionize as a predominantly self-employed workforce.[12] One of the main requests from participants was help gaining a better understanding of our rights and legal protections. In order for the union to provide this, we have to know what our worker status is, and this has proved to be incredibly complicated.

As it stands, the legal categorization of worker status within the UK is as shown in Table 15.1.

Unlike the US, the UK has an intermediary worker status, otherwise known as the 'limb (b)' category. This intermediary status has been instrumental in creating avenues and space for otherwise unrecognized self-employed workers to collectivize, acquire worker status, and, in doing so, reclaim rights and pay that they've been entitled to all along.

Amber Husain captures the neoliberal pitfalls of current employment law succinctly in *Replace Me* (2021):

> According to the UK's Employment Rights Act of 1996, 'no employment relationship exists if a worker can substitute another person to do the work'. This has been exploited – beneath a veneer of 'innovation' – by businesses in which inherently replaceable workers serve platforms rather than employers, and therefore forego the (already shrinking) rights afforded to full employees.
>
> Within this context...the less fortunate casual worker...misses out on sick pay, holiday pay, parental leave or protection from injustice at the hands of those by whom they aren't employed but for whom they nevertheless work.[13]

The IWGB, to which the Yoga Teachers Union is affiliated, is a small, independent, grassroot, and migrant-led trade union that has successfully and with renowned tenacity organized casual workers in multiple industries. One key landmark case that has effectively recategorized and therefore improved the working conditions and rights of gig economy workers is Aslam v Uber, 2021,[14] in which the UK Supreme Court held that Uber must pay its drivers the national minimum wage and at least 28 days paid holiday.

Yoga teachers are clearly encountering work patterns and challenges similar to that of the Uber drivers, and if we utilize similar organizing tactics it is highly likely that should a similar tribunal arise within our own industry, yoga teachers' status in many settings would be recategorized, affording them similar rights.

Table 15.1 RSA Gig Economy Chart[15]

	Self-Employed		Employee	
	Self-Employed	Worker (Limb-B worker)	Agency Worker	Employee
Legal Employment Status (in accordance with UK gig economy)	Also known as independent contractor, freelancer, or micro-entrepreneur. A person is self-employed if they are in business for themselves and enter into contracts with clients or customers to provide work or services for them.	Also known as 'limb (b) worker' and can be understood as a 'dependent contractor'. A 'worker' is registered as self-employed, but provides a service as part of someone else's business. They generally must carry out the work personally, rather than being able to send someone in their place. Their contract is not with their own client or customer, but with another party (i.e. a platform).	Generally, an agency worker has a contract with an agency, but works temporarily for a 'hirer' – a person or company with employees. After 12 weeks, they are entitled to the same rights as employees of the hiring company, but it is the agency that is responsible for their pay and administering statutory employment rights.	There is no universal definition of an employee in the UK, but an employee is understood to be a person who is contracted directly by a company. The employee will work to the terms within an employment contract (i.e. agreed pay, annual leave, and working hours), and will carry out the work personally.

Rights Under Employment Law

Employment law doesn't cover self-employed people in most cases because they are in business for themselves (i.e. their own boss). However, if a person is self-employed: • They still have protection for their health and safety and, in some cases, protection against discrimination. • Their rights and responsibilities are set out by the terms of the contract they have with their client.	• At least the National Minimum Wage • Protection against unlawful deductions from wages • Statutory minimum level of paid holiday • Statutory minimum length of rest breaks • Not obliged to work more than 48 hours on average per week, or to opt out of this right if they choose • Protection against unlawful discrimination • Protection for 'whistleblowing' (reporting wrongdoing in the workplace) • Equal treatment if working part-time.	From Day 1, an agency worker has the same rights as those in the 'worker' category. Additionally, agency workers have the same rights as colleagues employed by the hiring organisation to access shared facilities and services (such as the canteen or work transport). From 12 weeks, an agency worker has the same rights as colleagues employed by the hiring organisation. However, the clock resets each time they start at a new place of work.	All of the rights that 'workers' have and: • Statutory Sick Pay • Statutory Maternity, Paternity, Adoption, and Shared Parental Leave and Pay • Statutory Redundancy Pay • Minimum notice periods if their employment will be ending (i.e. if an employer is dismissing them) • Protection against unfair dismissal • The right to request flexible working • Time off for emergencies Some of these rights require a minimum length of continuous employment before an employee qualifies for them. An employment contract may state how long this qualification period is.

A recent New Economics Foundation (NEF) report, *Beyond the Gig Economy: Empowering the Self-Employed Workforce*, did acknowledge that despite the importance of accurately recategorizing worker status in this way, stamping out bogus self-employment in platform work doesn't go far enough.[16] Female-dominated precarious workforces have added issues to be addressed, and like many female-dominated precarious workforces, yoga teaching has an endemic problem with sexual abuse and harassment.

According to the NEF report, there has been a significant increase in the number of self-employed workers, which prior to the onset of the pandemic accounted for approximately 15 per cent of the UK's workforce (5 million people). There has been a specific increase in women and non-binary workers turning to self-employment:

> The erosion of standards, such as security over hours and pay, that has taken place in traditional forms of work in recent years, is likely to be a driver of self-employment growth. As an attractive alternative, self-employment is a form of work with the potential to provide an escape from some of the most damaging and oppressive elements of the traditional workplace. As such, it appeals to those who are most at risk of these oppressions, including women and migrant workers.[17]

This analysis strongly correlates with union members' reasons for becoming self-employed. Yoga teachers can be reluctant to unionize in case it means a return to the same employment structures that so many of us have consciously disengaged from. It's worth reassuring you that when unions successfully tackle bogus self-employment, workers are granted the rights they are already entitled to *without changing current working arrangements*. It is the miscategorization of yoga teachers' work that is being challenged, not the way in which you structure your work.

In working towards this goal, the Yoga Teachers Union is following in the footsteps of couriers and foster care workers before us. However, it is also clear that feminized workforces are woefully misunderstood by traditional union leadership. Diemet Bebuck rightfully questions this absence of understanding by union leadership:

> Looking specifically at the above-quoted UN statistic which indicates women's collective high work burdens and appallingly low control of material benefits, it is all the more astounding that materialist theorists have not been more forthcoming with discussions of the exploitation of women.[18]

As the NEF report shows, many have left traditional employment work structures due to discrimination, harassment, and abuse, or in the search for more supportive work hours to accommodate care needs, disabilities, and family responsibilities, and yet the self-employed status is more precarious, making workers more vulnerable and increasingly susceptible to discrimination, exploitation, and violence, whilst at the same time being less protected by employment law.

In order to organize effectively and make real change, it feels increasingly evident that we have to incorporate creativity and care, and recognize that whilst we can learn so much from the successful campaigns and legal battles of our fellow male-dominated branches, how we organize also needs to be different from what's come before us. When members sign up to the union, we ask them to select their reasons for joining. Achieving a living wage was third, at 67 per cent, behind addressing precarity (90 per cent) and becoming a part of a community (87 per cent). There is strength in numbers, and there is strength in connection and community. Sarah Jaffe states:

> Labour, after all, is us: messy, desiring, hungry, lonely, angry, frustrated human beings. We may be free to quit our jobs and find ones that we like better, as the mantra goes, but in practice that freedom is constrained by our need to eat, to have someplace to sleep, to have health care. Our place in the hierarchy of capitalist society is decided not by how hard we work but by any number of elements out of our control, including race, gender and nationality.[19]

After painting quite a bleak and overwhelming picture, it may come as a surprise that I'm actually filled with great hope and determination. Given the growth of precarious workers in feminized industries, and the gradual shift away from 'love and light' yoga towards an understanding of yoga teachers being workers, it is clear that there is a profound opportunity here. The more of us who organize, and the more we encourage and support each other in doing so, the more likely we are to shift these power dynamics and create alternatives that can break this cycle of exploitation and worker oppression. In one of our earliest strategy meetings, where attendance was high and energies were focused, we took some time, closed our eyes, and explored what our working lives *could* be. Even writing about it now, the hairs on the back of my neck stand up, and I can feel tears burning the back of my eyes. We collectively dared to imagine what our working lives could be with a sustainable income and holiday and sick pay. We imagined what it would be like to feel safe in our work and at work. It takes huge amounts of courage, persistence, and emotional strength to play a part in creating change, and to keep showing up in these spaces. The barriers and resistance are immense, but with each day that passes, we take an incremental step closer to bridging the gap between what is and what could be.

16 —

BRIGHTON YOGA FESTIVAL

Davy Jones

Davy Jones has been practising yoga since 1999 and teaching since 2007. In 2015, he was the first qualified yoga teacher to stand for parliament (for the Green Party in Brighton Kemptown). He co-founded the annual Brighton Yoga Festival which first took place in 2014 and set up the Brighton Yoga Foundation in 2016, which now runs the annual festival and coordinates programmes of community outreach yoga for those who would not normally have access to it. Prior to that, Davy was a political activist and campaigner and worked in public services for 30 years. He has two daughters from a previous relationship, and is now married to Janaki, a yoga teacher and co-organizer of yoga workshops and holidays under the auspices of InspirationYoga. He recently reached the ripe old age of 70 and wishes us to know that he still has his own teeth!

If Laura's chapter was a much-needed, sober account of money and power in yoga teaching, both Davy's chapter and the one that follows from Jivana Heyman are potential messages of hope. Like Laura and many of our contributors, Davy is clear about the disconnect between yoga teaching at the grassroots level, and yoga as a commercial industry. But Davy has a long and successful history of balancing these two aspects to the benefit of teachers and students alike. We asked him to tell us the story of Brighton Yoga Festival, sharing the positives and the negatives, the missed chances, and the moments of serendipity, as a case study. The result, once again, isn't a simple how-to guide for running a yoga charity. Instead, it is a glimpse into life of hard work and uneasy compromises, of authentic relationships and leveraging privilege to a greater good. This is, perhaps, what yoga teaching can be, if we are lucky.

They say money makes the world go round. And in our (capitalist) economic system, that is undoubtedly the case. The yoga community is not a separate 'all love and light' bubble, immune to that system and all its associated problems, especially when we consider who has the money and the power it confers. The growing commercialization of yoga, the increasing dominance of large chains of studios, the sexual abuse scandals in almost every yoga tradition, and the increasing recognition of the yoga community's lack of diversity are all stark reminders of how yoga suffers from similar problems to the rest of society.

According to published statistics, there are now as many as 300 million people regularly practising yoga around the world, and the yoga business is allegedly worth around £75 billion a year[1] – though the majority of yoga teachers get a very small slice of it! It is not surprising therefore that large corporations see huge opportunities to make a profit associated with yoga. Outside of the big cities in the UK in particular, yoga may still be practised in a local church or community hall with a local teacher charging very reasonable rates and teaching a range of philosophy, meditation, *prāṇāyāma*, and *āsana*. But this is rapidly changing, especially in the bigger cities, with big chains of yoga studios moving in to replace the local independent owners who generally saw providing yoga as a vocation and rarely made much money from it. Classes are being shortened, focused on *āsana*, and increasingly delivered by in-house and inadequately trained teachers.

There is a growing divergence in the yoga community internationally. If we simplify and generalize these changes, two broad trends are clear. On the one hand, there is an increasingly commercial strand to yoga, catering to individualistic ambitions – students in such classes often want to be fitter, and thus more attractive. The yoga that is so visible on Instagram feeds is delivered in gyms and yoga studio chains, and sustained by celebrity yoga teachers running huge workshops to maximize their income. There is limited interest in the history, philosophy, or ethics of yoga and usually little interest in sharing the benefits of the practice to those who need them most.

On the other hand is community yoga. This strand recognizes that personal liberation is inseparable from social liberation. It understands that yoga is rooted in society and should be committed to helping to solve its problems. It is less interested in hoarding knowledge for itself and is committed to using that knowledge and skill to help others. It sees yoga as potentially a major contributor towards general public health and well-being. This is particularly vital since the Covid-19 pandemic worsened mental health and respiratory and other ill-health conditions for many people.

Here in the city of Brighton & Hove, these two kinds of yoga overlap but they are still distinct. In 2022 there were around 20 local yoga studios, and dozens of gyms and community centres also providing regular classes. Across the rest of Sussex there were around 25 more yoga studios.[2] The vast majority were independent local businesses. Unless they are extremely wealthy, their owners have to make a profit from their studio to survive. Yet at the same time their ethos is usually generous, wanting to spread the benefits of yoga to others. They often joke to me about how they 'wear two hats – a yoga one, and a business one'. The two sit uneasily – as any two hats do on a single head! This can lead to tensions and rivalries between studios.

Studio owners spend a disproportionate amount of time and money on overheads, maintenance, and keeping their accounts in order: 'I spend more time fixing the boiler than I do teaching', one told me. Few of them make any profit. A tiny proportion are charities or community interest companies (CICs).

Anecdotally, most yoga studios locally (and elsewhere too) lost the majority of their regular members in the Covid-19 pandemic. The proliferation of online yoga (much of it free) had a huge impact on income. Some high-profile studios elsewhere in the country closed. Many teetered on the brink throughout the pandemic. With an ongoing financial crisis, as yet, the numbers of students attending classes remain stubbornly lower than in pre-pandemic days. Some studios will not survive. Those that do so are likely to have to increase their prices to make ends meet, making yoga even less accessible to those on low incomes. Inequality and relative poverty significantly affect who can access high-quality yoga teaching. For those outside the average yoga demographic, these barriers reinforce the image of yoga as being 'not for ordinary people like me'.

Increasingly, organizations such as Move GB or MindBodyOnline have moved in to take a slice of the yoga industry, providing clients and booking and payment systems to allow teachers to focus on teaching rather than administration. But this comes at a hefty price and reduces the income of studio owners and teachers alike. Fortunately, other booking systems that are developed and run by yoga teachers do exist (e.g. Reservie: www.reservie.net).

We have hundreds of yoga teachers in Brighton & Hove,[3] probably the highest number per head of population of anywhere in the UK, maybe even in Europe. A significant proportion of those do not teach regularly. The truth is that it is very hard to make a living as a yoga teacher unless you reach 'celebrity status' and can run large workshops here and abroad, teach on prestigious yoga teacher training courses, and/or write yoga books.[i] Most local yoga teachers supplement the small income they receive from yoga teaching with at least one 'proper job'. The yoga teacher training juggernaut keeps producing ever more teachers, which makes it even harder to make a living. Few such courses include sessions on ethical business standards or reference how hard it is to make a living from yoga teacher training.

Meanwhile, pay increases for yoga teachers in gyms and studios are rare – some teachers report receiving the same amount per class as when they started 10 or even 20 years ago. Many teachers see teaching as a vocation and feel under pressure to provide access to the practice for free or very cheaply. Often teachers are driven to take on punishing schedules of classes to make ends meet. When they do so, yoga teaching becomes a lot like other forms of alienating work, and such teachers risk burnout. The power relations between studios and teachers are often brutal. There is little transparency about who is paid what and where the money goes. No wonder there is increasing interest in the Independent Workers Union of Great Britain (IWGB) Yoga Teachers Union.

THE YOGA FESTIVAL BEGINNINGS
Brighton Yoga Foundation (BYF; www.brightonyogafoundation.org) has an interesting history, which has been consistently intertwined with political, ethical, and financial issues.

In late 2013, I was selected by the Brighton & Hove Green Party to be its parliamentary candidate for the 2015 general election in the Kemptown constituency. It was a marginal seat between Labour and Conservatives, and in those days the Greens were a long way behind with no realistic chance of winning.

I did a bit of research and discovered that I was the first fully qualified yoga teacher to stand for parliament in the UK! I thought that fact was pretty funny and something that I could use in my election campaign. So, I contacted a number of friends and teachers in the yoga community and we began organizing to stage the first ever Brighton Yoga Festival for a Saturday in July 2014 in the Kemptown constituency in the run-up to the 2015 general election.

Brighton & Hove is a small city with less than 300,000 people. But it has

---

i   The editors of this text recognize the irony of this point and would like to point out that you don't get much for writing books either!

arguably the biggest yoga community in the UK, if not Europe, as a proportion of its population. So, while there had been other yoga festivals around the UK before 2014, it was surprising that Brighton & Hove had not already held one.

From the outset, we wanted to attract the maximum number of people to the event who had never tried yoga before. We found a church in Kemptown with a wonderful large space, some additional side-rooms, and a small outside area, costing just a few hundred pounds. That gave us the confidence to announce that the festival would be free (while welcoming donations!). We also agreed to have collection buckets for two local Kemptown charities (one for older people, the other for the local centre for the unemployed).

We asked local teachers to teach for free at the event, in return for us promoting their involvement. We found a yoga studio to sponsor the event, sold food and retail franchises, and overall managed to balance the £2500 expenditure with a similar income, as well as raising a few hundred pounds for the local charities. We got our local (Green) MP Caroline Lucas to open the event. In addition, I delivered a talk on yoga and politics. I began wearing a suit and a bowler hat and a briefcase and gradually stripped off into my yoga clothes. Throughout the talk I moved through various yoga postures, all the while musing on the inter-relationship between politics and yoga![4] We had hoped for an attendance of around 500 overall but 1200 people came. The following year at the same venue we had 1800 people attending.

Looking back on those early financial decisions, in truth I am not sure we realized just how bold and unusual that approach was to staging a yoga festival. Since then, we have looked at many other yoga events both here and abroad and almost all of them charge a significant entry fee in order to cover their costs. That is an entirely understandable and legitimate approach. But it does of course mean that it is likely to attract only the existing yoga community and those who have sufficient disposable income to pay the entrance charge.

The Brighton Yoga Festival has continued every year since. The numbers attending grew and stabilized for 2016–2019 at between 2500 and 3000 people. We expanded the festival from one day to a whole summer weekend in the years from 2017 to 2020. The overall budget for the event crept up to just under £20,000. Then in 2020 and 2021, the festival moved online due to the pandemic, and contracted in numbers and scope.

The festival is no longer associated with the Green Party or seen as a party-political event, though we have taken environmental, ethical, and political stances on a number of issues: only serving vegetarian or vegan food and drinks; banning single-use plastics; and not having mainstream sponsors or retailers whose ethics we felt uncomfortable including in the yoga world.

We have also regularly addressed controversial and political issues, staging a solidarity event of yogis for Extinction Rebellion and a survivor-led panel on the sexual abuse crisis in the yoga community (both in 2019), a panel of black yoga activists on Black Lives Matter and the lack of diversity in yoga (2020), and a session on the future of yoga post-pandemic and promoting the new yoga teachers trade union (2021). This stance hasn't always proved popular with everyone. But we believe that yoga and politics cannot be kept separate and that yoga philosophy itself encourages ethical, inclusive, and progressive approaches to societal issues.

Throughout the years of the festival being free to attend, we sought sponsors, sold food and retail franchises, and vigorously fundraised at the events themselves. Anecdotally, we noticed that the people who were happy to buy expensive yoga leggings at the retail stalls tended to be the least generous at donating to the collection buckets! On the other hand, some people (including less well-off participants) stuffed £20 notes into our collecting buckets saying that it had been a wonderful occasion. We sold programmes for £1 or £2 to raise additional money and encountered resistance from many festival-goers with comments like 'We thought this was a free event.' It opened our eyes to the massive diversity of opinions and experiences in the yoga community on financial matters.

Since 2019 our annual festival has been financed on the *dana* (giving or gift) principle of 'pay what you can afford'. This model has been challenging. In the first year of this approach – 2019 – well over half of the people who registered to attend the festival paid nothing! We are not sure why. Perhaps we didn't explain the model clearly enough or explain that the festival was designed to raise money for our yoga outreach work. Perhaps they were used to it being free in previous years and didn't really understand the new model. Perhaps some of those who did not pay when registering were amongst those who donated generously when they subsequently attended the festival in person. But such a high proportion was completely unexpected, and frankly disappointing. We had expected to receive well over £10,000 in advance registrations online but our actual total was around £6500.

In 2020 the festival had to be online due to Covid-19 and the online sessions were also publicised as 'pay what you can afford'. But this time we explained more clearly how the funds raised would be used, and gave a recommended donation of £20 for each two-hour workshop session. This time only around 20 per cent donated nothing and we received donations from

£1 to £100, with an average of just under £20 per person. The event overall made a profit that we ploughed into our yoga outreach work.

We have investigated other paid-for models of running the festival. We believe that charging a commercial rate for the event would lead to a drastic reduction in the numbers of those attending. In turn, that would mean that the sponsors, retailers, and food and drink providers would get far less publicity and sales, and would only be willing to pay a much lower sponsorship or franchise fee than for the previous bigger events. We would also then be ethically obliged to pay teachers for their involvement. Up to now we have always asked teachers if they would be prepared to teach in return for travel expenses, as an act of solidarity with the foundation's charitable aims and projects.

Surprisingly, when we modelled the various options available, we found that the overall balance between projected income and expenditure for the event was roughly similar whether it was pay what you can afford or a normal commercial rate. It seems self-evident therefore to persevere with the pay what you can afford model, despite the challenges.

BECOMING A CHARITY

After the second annual yoga festival in 2015, we began to discuss our vision of bringing the benefits of yoga to those who don't normally have access to it. While the two festivals had been very successful, it was clear that they were not attracting a significantly new demographic. We became a registered charity (a CIO or charitable incorporated organization) in May 2016. We followed the tried and tested community development principle: to go out to the communities we wished to reach, instead of expecting them to come to our events.

At the start, we had accumulated a small sum (£1000) and advertised for people with innovative ideas for yoga projects to apply for funding. We agreed to fund three short local projects – an LGBT young people's yoga class, another for women recovering from depression, and one bringing nursery children and elderly care home residents together into a yoga class. They were all successful. But we decided in the end that we would rather organize our community outreach work ourselves.

Our first issue was how to fund the community outreach yoga programmes that we wanted to run. A ten-week course of classes would typically cost around £1500. Sometimes the class needed to be in a specific location and we had to pay a commercial rate for the hire. For other classes, we approached local yoga studios. Some offered us a space for free, others at cheap rates if we organized the classes in quiet periods of their schedules.

We took the decision early on to pay the teachers delivering these outreach courses a proper commercial rate (approx. £40 for a one-hour class). All our teachers have undergone specialist advanced yoga training and we felt they should be rewarded accordingly for teaching.

Without any rich benefactors or other sources of income, and with the early festivals only breaking even financially, it soon became apparent that the most effective way of funding the proposed outreach classes was through grants. Between the start of 2017 and the summer of 2022, we made 42 grant applications. Some 26 applications were successful, raising just over £100,000.

Writing grant applications takes a lot of time and skill. We were fortunate to get advice from two local experts in this field who were supportive of our work. Being successful in the applications gave us a huge boost. But it is only then that the work starts. Most funders have very specific conditions and strict monitoring requirements. Failing to provide monitoring reports effectively prevents any follow-up applications. Our experience is that if you follow their processes, funding bodies are very supportive and pragmatic. On occasions, we have been forced (especially during the pandemic) to significantly alter what we promised to deliver in the original application. In every case when we have contacted the funders and explained our reasons carefully, they have approved our changes.

We have been fortunate to receive modest but consistent support from Brighton & Hove Council, including funds to help cover some of our core administrative and running costs. This is unusual as most funders only support specific projects. A regional funding umbrella body (Sussex Community Foundation) has also funded a number of our projects. We have had mixed fortunes dealing with the National Lottery and its various funding streams. But perhaps the biggest surprise has been the amount of funds that we have received from regional and national sporting bodies – Active Sussex and Sport England. They have been particularly supportive of any projects that we proposed for women, ethnic minorities, and young people.

At the time of writing, we have 12 weekly outreach classes running or about to start, with more than 100 people attending a class each week. The classes are all provided free of charge to remove any financial barrier to participants' involvement. But we do encourage (and sometimes receive) donations from some of those who are in a position to contribute. There is a considerable amount of organization and coordination involved in such a programme, especially as many of the participants in the classes need a lot of support and pastoral care. We have managed to include an element in most of our grant applications that covers the costs of someone to coordinate the work. But as we have seized every opportunity to expand the programme of classes, we are constantly playing catch-up with the scale of time and resources needed to coordinate them.

We have also tried to develop a national network of yoga organizations with a similar ethos and approach to providing community yoga outreach to those who need it. We have been inspired in particular by the work and history of Edinburgh Community Yoga. But partly due to Covid and the pressures on local yoga groups, we have not made as much progress as we had hoped. We are also keen to link up with similar organizations internationally, such as Accessible Yoga and similar movements in the USA.

As of yet, the Brighton Yoga Foundation has no full-time staff or even an office (though it does rent a space for storage of all our equipment – mostly for the festivals). We have employed a part-time outreach programmes coordinator and a freelance accountant, a marketing/social media person, and a manager for our annual festival. We really need a full-time director or chief executive post. Without it, our trustees have to combine their strategic role of leading the charity with day-to-day delivery and organizational work. This puts an excessive demand on our trustees, and has led to burnout. Finding a funding body that can finance such a role is rare. Applications are fiercely competitive and so far, we have been unsuccessful.

It is important to acknowledge that some yoga teachers have been doing this type of outreach yoga for some time, usually without making a fuss about it or seeking any recognition. The same is true of yoga in schools. Many primary schools in our city (and elsewhere) had been pioneering the benefits of yoga for young people long before we got involved. We see our role as a yoga charity in promoting that work and making it consistently available for all those who need it. We have also encouraged all the yoga studios in the city to provide free or cheap community classes, and many now do so.

We have tried other fundraising techniques. We have been very lucky to receive significant financial support and encouragement from Yogamatters, the UK's largest supplier of yoga equipment. We were included for a number of years in their High Fives programme supporting organizations involved in community yoga outreach. They also generously donated 250 yoga mats to us for use at our annual festivals, saving us high rental fees for the yoga mats that we need each year. But we have been very cautious about agreeing to other commercial sponsorship (not that there have been many offers!). We do not want to be associated with any companies or organizations whose ethics and behaviour are not aligned with our own. Arguably this 'cuts off our nose to spite our face' but we couldn't bring ourselves to be promoting companies or products that we felt uncomfortable with. For that reason, we have been reluctant to seek support from corporate entities such as Lululemon, which operate charitable funds for yoga outreach projects, though we are aware that other like-minded yoga organizations have found that to be fruitful. We may be revisiting that issue in the near future as a local branch has just opened in Brighton!

We have tried other fundraising routes, such as selling merchandise. This didn't prove successful without a permanent outlet to sell the products. We have received one legacy following the passing of a local yoga teacher and we are now investigating how to make that an ongoing source of income. Without being morbid, quite a few experienced yoga teachers (myself included!) are now in the 'late autumn' of their lives and may wish to support the yoga community in perpetuity. We have also set up the Friends of Brighton Yoga Foundation to provide a future source of income and volunteers for our work. Friends will be expected either to donate regularly via direct debit and/or, for those unable to donate, to promise a number of hours of voluntary time per month.

CONCLUDING THOUGHTS

Looking back at this journey, it is striking to me how few of the issues that we have encountered were envisaged at the beginning. It all seemed so simple: 'Let's organize a yoga festival and bring yoga to those who can't access it.' What could possibly go wrong or be difficult about that?

We have learnt a lot about organization, networking, and building teams and alliances. Above all we have spent a lot of time worrying about money! It is relatively easy to provide one-off classes or small events for free, drawing on the goodwill of yoga teachers. But ongoing programmes or courses require money – for the teacher, the venue, equipment, publicity, and for someone to organize them. There is simply no getting away from it. We have tried to approach every issue concerning money from an ethical perspective – not just because we are a charity, but because we want to be true to our beliefs and to our approach to yoga. Arguably it is harder – but we feel better and truer to our values for doing so. Others will have to judge whether we have made the right decisions or not.

None of us started this process to make money – which in hindsight is just as well. We had a passion about the value and benefits of yoga and how those who would arguably benefit the most were those who did not have easy access to it. The impact of the Covid-19 pandemic has only reinforced that belief.

Brighton Yoga Foundation is now an established and credible organization. But to be truly sustainable, and to expand its work any further, we would need to take its infrastructure to a whole new level, with a manager, an office, and perhaps other part-time staff. And that requires even more money![i] Of course, that will mean we take on more responsibilities and start to wear those two hats I spoke about at the start – more ethical dilemmas.

Since I started writing this piece, perhaps the most prestigious yoga chain in London, Triyoga, has been taken over by a hedge fund,[5] one of the biggest yoga teacher training organizations, YogaLondon, has gone into voluntary liquidation,[6] and locally, the Brighton Natural Health Centre, which has been offering yoga for 42 years, has had to close its building (though it hopes to relaunch itself in a new location in 2023). Yet the need for yoga and the benefits it brings have never been greater. As I write this conclusion, cities across Ukraine are being bombed and innocent people are dying in their hundreds. And the latest Inter-Governmental Panel on Climate Change (IPCC) report is the starkest yet about the risks to the human race if we do not more rapidly tackle climate change.[7]

The yoga world is not immune to and cannot ignore the huge environmental, political, and socio-economic issues we all face. And it has to face those external issues and its own internal issues using the core of yoga philosophy:

- *ahiṃsā*, non-violence to oneself or others
- *satya*, truth and transparency
- *asteya*, non-stealing from others (including future generations)
- *aparigraha*, generosity and non-greed.

Yoga should be about making the world a better place.

---

i   Feel free to send large donations!

17 —

JIVANA'S HOMEWORK

Jivana Heyman

Jivana Heyman (he/him), is the author of *Accessible Yoga: Poses and Practices for Every Body* (2019), and *Yoga Revolution: Building a Practice of Courage and Compassion* (2021).[1] Jivana is the founder and director of the Accessible Yoga Association, an international non-profit organization dedicated to increasing access to the yoga teachings. He's also the co-founder of the Accessible Yoga School, an online portal focusing on equity and accessibility.

Like Davy, Jivana has a history of playing the uncomfortable boundary between the interests of industry and social justice in yoga, to the benefit of the latter. We've known Jivana for a long time, in fact, we (Harriet and Theo) met him at the first Accessible Yoga conference in Europe, and became instant co-conspirators there. During the conference, Jivana talked openly about having been approached by the clothing mega-brand, Lululemon, with an offer of financial support for his work. The resulting debate was polarizing but good-natured, but we were mostly impressed by Jivana's willingness to discuss and take the community's advice about funding issues that most yoga charities decide in private.

We asked Jivana, like Davy, for a chapter about power and money in the inevitable business politics that emerge when you run a non-profit organization on an international scale. Like most similar charities, no matter the scale of the sums involved, the numbers of people actually running these organizations are small. In this piece, Jivana offers a more personal reflection on using some of the teachings of yoga philosophy to frame our interactions with money and power. He emphasizes the importance of relationship and community, above that of individual branding and the demands of the wellness industry. Most of all, this chapter demonstrates how opening yourself up to the relationship between money and power in yoga leaves you with more questions than answers. His conclusion, and ours, is that leaning into these questions with an attitude of openness, non-attachment, service, and community is the only way for change to happen. It is a conclusion that Davy and Laura would agree with.

We know yoga teachers struggle to make a living wage, and we often talk among ourselves about the complex role of money in yoga. But what I don't think we talk about enough is the role of power, not only how power is at the heart of yoga business and culture, but how the teachings of yoga place power at the very heart of yoga practice and philosophy.

Of course, yoga has many meanings and such a rich and diverse history. Its practice and teaching are interpreted in many ways, and I can only share from my own perspective. After over 30 years of practice, I'm always learning and expanding my knowledge of that which is not easily defined.

I see the issue of power reflected in what I consider to be the most important teaching in yoga: the idea that all we seek exists within us as our most essential Self. From this perspective, our spirit, *puruṣa* or *atman*, is completely free and unaffected by anything in the external world. This unchanging, immortal part of us never changes, even though our body and mind are constantly changing. This is the source of all happiness, joy, fulfilment, and indeed power.

In short, as I see it, clearly our practice is about remembering this essential truth, and uncovering the power that lays dormant within us. In the *Chandogya Upanishad*, which is over 2500 years old, there is a beautiful section that speaks to the power we have within:

> The little space within the heart is as great as this vast universe. The heavens and the earth are there, and the sun, and the moon, and the stars; fire and lightning and winds are there; and all that now is and all that is not: for the whole universe is in Him and He dwells within our heart.[2]

I love the idea that we have the whole universe in the little space within our heart, mostly because I often feel the exact opposite. I struggle with anxiety, constantly comparing myself to others, questioning myself and my self-worth. So, the idea that this tremendous source of power resides within my own heart is a revelation to me.

This concept also reminds me of similar teachings in the *Yoga Sūtra of Patañjali*: that I have all I need within. Patañjali simply calls it non-attachment, which many translators define as freedom from selfish desire. But, if you think about it, freedom from selfish desire occurs when we realize that we are already fulfilled, that we already have all that we need inside.

This inner resource, or inner power, is in direct opposition to the core principle of capitalism, which teaches us that we need to earn, buy, and achieve our way to happiness or worthiness. Our self-doubt is used against us by a system that is designed for profit-making. Any time we're feeling insecure, author Sonya Renee Taylor recommends that we ask ourselves, 'Who is profiting off my insecurity?'[3]

The sheer beauty, and dare I say power, of yoga is that it begins with this completely radical notion that we are full, fine, and whole, from the moment we are born to the moment that we die. As Patañjali explains:

> Nonattachment is the manifestation of self-mastery in one who is free from craving for objects seen or heard about. When there is non-thirst for even the gunas (constituents of nature) due to realization of the Purusha, that is supreme nonattachment. (1.15–1.16)[4]

Most yoga teachers know that the commercial yoga industry is focused on hoarding power and money. It is easy therefore for us to demonize that business world as something separate and other, as if we are not a part of it. Instead, it can be useful to consider the ways in which the world is really a reflection of our own ego-mind. In so many ways, this grasping industry is just like my mind, which also clings to the belief that external things will make me happy. So as a yoga teacher, am I participating in and perpetuating a yoga culture also based on this misapprehension? This leads me to ask: Is it even possible to practice and teach in a way that honors the yoga teachings that I feel are essential? If so, what would that look like?

To be honest, I don't think it would look anything like what we see in the yoga world today. Perhaps a yoga culture built to reflect the teachings themselves. A yoga world built on *ahiṃsā*, or *seva*, would be different not only in its outer appearance, but also in terms of content – what is shared – and methodology – how it's shared.

The yoga teachings above call for a radical shift in our understanding of our relationship to each other. While some yoga teachings are about abandoning the world, there are others, like in the *Bhagavad Gītā*, that teach us that we are all connected. In the end, 'community' is the word that best speaks to the message of these yoga teachings, but it fails to express the many ways in which we are all intimately connected. My heart is the same as yours, but is it my heart that guides my decision-making, or is my ego-mind still looking to get or achieve something in order to be fulfilled?

The power of culture, language, and capitalism are all focused on elevating the individual above the masses. In the *Gītā*, Kṛṣṇa clearly says that enlightenment is not only seeing the divine in everything, but it is literally feeling the pleasure and pain of others as our own:

> As your mind becomes harmonized through yoga practices, you begin to see the atman in all beings and all beings in your Self: you see the same Self everywhere and in everything. The yogi who perceives the essential oneness everywhere naturally feels the pleasure or pain of others as his or her own. (6.29–32)[5]

Unfortunately, even as capitalism tempts us to look outward for fulfilment and happiness, it also puts the burden of caring for ourselves back on our own shoulders and calls it 'self-care'. We're caught in a double bind – needing to achieve outward success and simultaneously needing to find our own inner peace. True self-care would be the ability to rest when needed, to have ample paid time off for illness, or to care for loved ones. This form of self-care is possible when our basic needs are met, which means that a healthy society ensures the basics of housing, food, and healthcare for all. True self-care is in fact community care. These aren't problems that a personal practice of meditation and *āsana* can solve alone.

Capitalism has packaged the ancient and Indigenous spiritual teachings of yoga into 'wellness', and left those among us who are most bereft of power to fend for ourselves under the guise of self-care. Rather than allowing us to care for each other, or create systems of community care, we are forced to go it alone. 'Every man for himself' is the message we are given over and over. This is most obvious within the international yoga industry. Here, physical achievement is seen as the highest form of success, even though many traditional practices of yoga focus on service to others as the key to our enlightenment.

Another major difference between these traditional teachings and the yoga industry is in the pursuit of celebrity and success by individual yoga teachers. It's ironic that in my efforts to teach and share yoga I find myself constantly asked to put myself forward as an individual teacher and personality, even though my goal has been to serve my community. Of course, my ego loves the attention, and so I'm torn between my ego's desire for power, and the higher calling of yoga to serve and love, and to share the message that yoga is there for all of us.

I often have to pause and ask myself: What is the goal of my practice? Is it personal enlightenment, or individual success? Is it even possible to achieve individual enlightenment if my community is struggling? In the end, isn't that what social justice is about: wanting justice for everyone; wanting everyone to have a chance to succeed, and for everyone to enjoy the same basic human rights?

I have tried to embody the intersection of yoga and social justice through the non-profit that I founded, the Accessible Yoga Association. Together we work to find ways to make yoga accessible outside of the mainstream and commercial yoga industry. Our emphasis has been on community building and mutual support among yoga teachers. This takes the form of educational and networking opportunities such as conferences and community forums.

At every one of our conferences, I challenge the participants to find somebody else at the event they can support in some way. I call this assignment #JivanasHomework, and I emphasize the importance of peer networking in creating a grassroots yoga movement that is not dependent on corporate interests. I encourage all attendees to either collaborate on a project with somebody else in attendance, or to lift them up in some way, even without them knowing. They could, for example, share about somebody else's work on social media. They could recommend someone for a job, or they could introduce someone to a colleague to help further their work. These kinds of peer support networks are incredibly effective for those of us who are working outside the corporate yoga industry.

But the irony of the non-profit yoga world is that we are still completely dependent on corporate interests. Accessible Yoga uses a membership model, but we also get grants from foundations and corporations.

In October 2018, as I was preparing for our first European Accessible Yoga Conference just outside of Berlin, I found out that Lululemon, the large multinational clothing company, was interested in giving us a large grant. It was exciting to think of all the programming we could do with a big chunk of money, but it was disturbing to consider the source of that funding. In particular, I could not ignore the way that Lululemon had harmed the yoga community through its overly competitive, ableist approach to marketing yoga as a lifestyle for the young, thin, and beautiful.

During a workshop at the conference, I took the opportunity to ask the attendees what they thought I should do: take the money or reject the money?

Just as I did, everyone there had very mixed feelings about it. Most people felt that we should take the money and use it for good, but there were a few clear voices of dissent who spoke to the dangers of selling out and becoming indebted to corporate interests. In the end, we took the money after clarifying with Lululemon that we had the freedom to spend it as we wanted to, and that we didn't need to promote them through our work.

Even though I struggled with taking their money, it has allowed us to continue our service these past few years. In fact, that Europe conference ended up being a bit of a financial disaster that left us in debt. Without the grant from Lululemon we would have had to fold. Instead, we've managed to move our conferences online, and expand our programming exponentially by adding monthly events and community forums. Most importantly, we have used grants, from Lululemon and others, to allow us to avoid the current online yoga summit model, which only pays presenters when they make affiliate sales. Instead, we are able to platform an incredibly diverse group of yoga teachers – and pay them for their time.

Over the years, I find these kinds of situations leave me with more questions than answers. Every step that we take as a participant in a system of capitalist oppression simply keeps that system churning. It is only when we are actively engaged in either dismantling it or creating alternative ways to be that we are being true to the yoga teachings. So that makes me think of more questions: how do you reconcile yoga, money, and power? Can you teach yoga in a way that interrupts the capitalist system and is a reflection of the yoga teachings? Can your practice and teaching be of service to yourself, your community, and to the entire world?

I don't have clear answers to these questions, but I believe that we need to keep asking them of ourselves and our colleagues. Within the questioning, and these conversations with colleagues, we can begin to imagine a new way of practicing and teaching that not only reflects the heart of the yoga teachings, but the innate power and agency of each individual teacher and practitioner.

CONCLUSION

What Keeps Us Up at Night

YOU'VE COME A LONG WAY, BABY

Looking back over the content of this book is quite a journey. From trauma to racism, labour relations to abuse, it is perhaps no wonder that so many yoga teachers face at least one crisis of confidence in their career. For us, Harriet and Theo, this book is the continuation of a thread that reaches back all the way to the first time we met, at the Accessible Yoga Europe Conference in 2018. What we shared then was a firm conviction that yoga teaching could be more inclusive, more equitable, more sustainable, and more strongly rooted in both science and history. We truly believed that yoga teaching could be all that, and still hold those moments of magic that made it all worthwhile.

Since that day, the pressure on yoga teachers has only increased, much of it due to forces far beyond the yoga world. As Laura Hancock reminds us, yoga teachers are part of a precarious workforce, and a caring and therapeutic profession. We are especially vulnerable to pandemic lockdowns, misinformation, health care crises, and cost of living increases.

Theo has been talking to people who, like Karin Carlson, have decided to move away from yoga teaching. They talk about difficulties adapting to teaching online during the COVID pandemic, personal illness, and injury. They talk about their frustration with cultural appropriation, spiritual bypassing, lack of fair pay, and a lack of recognition for their training and experience. It is obvious to us that many of us who are still yoga teachers share the same concerns, and many of the same experiences.

Yet of all the 'ex' yoga teachers who are taking part in Theo's research, very few say they will never teach yoga again. There's something about being a yoga teacher that casts a long shadow, and etches a groove in your identity.

The people in this book are also not ready to give up on the potential of this complex and contradictory practice.

Some of you will reach this point and gain the momentum you need to teach less or not at all. Others will reach this point having gathered the resources to start new yoga teaching projects. Either way, we hope this book is a blessing to you. We do, however, encourage you to arrange your working lives to include more than yoga teaching, if you can. Harriet and Theo both teach a little yoga, we train yoga teachers a lot, and we both work for other people, teaching, writing, researching, even baking. Not everything in life can be sustained by yoga alone.

What sustains us is the relationships that we in turn sustain. What has been variously described in this book as communities of practice, beloved communities, and circles of trust is a key theme for many of our writers. As we said in our introduction, these are just some of the people that we choose to work with. But as Jivana's homework reminds us, these relationships of collaboration, of co-conspiracy, of friendship, and even of altruism, are built on so much more than cold calculations about networking and shared reach on social media. They are built on more than yoga too.

The real question here is: who can you work with and how do you work with them? Who do you trust? Who do you run to when you're processing yet another guru accusation, or the latest research? How do we support each other when so many of the issues, and so much of the trauma in yoga, is coming from other yoga teachers? Who will you be seen sharing a platform with?

WALKING OUT

We started this book by talking about bad yoga teaching. We have never meant to malign yoga teachers when we say that. In our experience, yoga teachers are, in the majority, well-meaning, thoughtful, lifelong learners. Yet the media aimed at yoga teachers, the trainings you are offered, and the books you are sold so often contain far too much misinformation. They also contain far too little pedagogy. In the main, yoga teacher trainings consist mostly of practice content (what to do in your practice) and instructional techniques (how to get students to do what you want them to). Beyond a few hours on the *yamas* and *niyamas*, the ethics and practice of teaching itself are rarely examined.

We believe that the 'why' of teaching is as important as the 'how'. Indeed, if you are not clear about the relationship between instruction, effect, and intention, you are arguably not teaching at all. The yoga industry trains yoga teachers in ever more refinements to describe and demonstrate standing up straight, without ever asking: does being shown how to stand up straight translate into standing up straight in daily life? And why are we teaching people that there is a right and a wrong way to stand at all?

One of the biggest lies you have been sold is that there could ever be one simple answer to such complex questions as how to teach inclusively, or what practices are 'good' or 'safe' for which students. Perhaps an even bigger lie is the idea that you, in your yoga class, can cure this or that condition; that yoga teaching is essential to anti-justice work; that you intuitively know more than doctors; and that you can hold a safe space for group therapy without further training and support. In fact, most yoga teachers reach a crisis of confidence when they first experience a gap between the instruction, effect, and intention of the practice. It is often at this point that they seek out further study in the practice and philosophy of pedagogy itself.

There is a special kind of relief that comes from releasing those overblown expectations about what a yoga teacher is capable of. Staying within your scope of practice is a safer space for you and your students-to-be. More than that, we encourage you to apply scepticism to the claims of those trying to sell you the answers to these impossible expectations. Encourage the same scepticism and questioning in your students. That is the foundation of a truly effective yoga pedagogy.

For many of the contributors to this book, leading trainings for yoga teachers involves a significant amount of debunking. Yet elsewhere, without naming names, there are well-respected authorities on yoga whose ways of working are still based on instruction rather than enquiry. Their methods do not change because yoga teachers, on the whole, are just a little too respectful of authority. As Theo is fond of asking yoga teachers: when was the last time you walked out of a workshop?

Here are just a few of the things that would make us walk out.

Justice by numbers

There is a strong tendency in social justice work to confuse the actual issue with the group identity of those affected. A justice-by-numbers approach to cultural appropriation, for example, treats any South Asian or diasporic teacher as an absolute authority on yoga. It fails to examine issues of gender and caste, and most often, serves to platform white guilt rather than provoke actual change. In this book, Sheena Sood speaks most eloquently to this effect, calling it 'Omwashing'.

Omwashing is common because actual change is hard, and implicates us in movements of solidarity that measure success in decades, not an afternoon workshop. There are many other examples of justice-focused workshops and trainings that focus on tribal politics and superficial analysis, and leave participants with a lot of guilt and very few pathways to effective change. We encourage you to sit with how such workshops make you feel. A sense of personal discomfort, anger, or grief is usual. A sense of impotence, rage, or shame is not.

Mob healing, mob justice

A very similar process of mis-application happens in many projects on spiritual abuse in yoga. It is alarmingly common to reduce this complex phenomenon to women as victims and men as aggressors, or worse, white women as victims of South Asian men. Not all the victims of spiritual abuse are women, nor are all abusers men. Many of the first or main victims of some of the most heinous crimes by charismatic yoga teachers have been South Asian. Among the few female charismatic yoga teachers, there are notable examples of insidious and long-term interpersonal, even sexual abuse.

Yet workshops on spiritual abuse commonly consist of circles of women vicariously re-traumatizing each other without therapeutic oversight or resolution. In reality, we need to address power imbalances between abusers and victims, and the relationships and structures that enable the abuse at a collective level, as the UK Yoga Teachers Union is attempting to do. But whenever you hear a leading authority in yoga refer to any contentious issue by a group identity or label, we encourage you to be cautious. Not 'all' trauma survivors hate to be touched in a yoga class. Not 'all' abusers are men. Not 'all' cis women share specific bodily experiences that trans women, any men, or non-binary people do not.

Justice fatigue and the urgency of training

Social media in particular has evolved less as a channel for information or social connection, and more as a contagion field for emotion and misinformation. We are all exhausted by the flood of calls on our time and attention for anything from school shootings in the US to wildfires in Europe and floods in East Asia. It is common practice now to market yoga teacher trainings and workshops with a similar sense of urgency. Yet if you know what you know (stay in your scope of practice) and don't over-promise, if you treat your students with respect and approach them with genuine curiosity, you have a good foundation on which to slowly, sustainably involve yourself in further study and training. There really is no rush, no hurry.

Communities of care are sites of resistance for many marginalized and oppressed populations. In many cases, our friends, colleagues, and siblings in the fight are the source of any healing or justice we might find. But circles of trauma survivors or the chronically ill are not on their own a recipe for healing, and gossip about which charismatic teachers are not 'safe' to be alone with are a poor substitute for justice. If you are involved in similar work, regularly ask yourself: how are your common causes being weaponized, against whom, and who profits from your frustration?

Citation as obfuscation

This next point is more difficult to address. Because yoga teachers are invested in authority (more on that in Theo's first book, *Post-Lineage Yoga*!) we have a strong tendency to use big names as talismans to reflect their authority back on ourselves. When, for example, a 'trauma-informed' yoga workshop claims to have based its material on 'polyvagal theory', that does not mean that the practices it will teach have been scientifically tested by Stephen Porges himself, *even if he did write the introduction to the manual.* They certainly won't have been subject to a major meta-analysis or even tested by multiple large-scale research projects. This simply isn't feasible.

Meanwhile, a great number of the 'translations' of Patañjali's *Yoga Sūtras* are in fact interpretations written by authors who are not Sanskrit scholars. Theo tries not to do web searches for 'post-lineage yoga', for fear of what misinformation is being spread in her name. And an MA in yoga and meditation studies from SOAS does not make anyone an expert in pre-modern yoga practice. Beware of anyone who can give you the 'truth' of history or science in a single book or a single course.

It is difficult for you, as a student at a workshop, to know if the people leading it are accurately representing the research or the philosophies or the ancient worldviews they are presenting to you. But citational politics and practice do matter. Where you can, we advise you to check the sources you are given, and if no source or reference is given, we suggest you might want to withdraw your participation.

F*cked up by yoga

Theo has a friend, Jude, who runs the most excellent podcast called 'Fkd up by faith'.[1] Jude once described this as 'being rejected by your faith community; rejecting your faith community; having a crisis of faith; realizing that you believe some things and not others; or disagreeing with your church or religious group's views'.

It is beyond time that we as yoga teachers reflect and share the times that we have all been 'f*cked up' by yoga. We aren't suggesting this as a means of tearing yoga down. As Barbora reminds us, 'yoga' is a term that has evolved almost beyond recognition, across thousands of years. It is bigger than whatever criticism we can throw at it. But an informed critique of established knowledge, and the regular testing of established practice is in fact how we make our practices better, and more robust.

In May 2022, Theo was diagnosed with an auto-immune condition. These days, her Twitter feed is full of disability activists and the chronically ill. The most common joke on those threads is 'have you tried yoga?' Outside of social media, multiple people have suggested various yoga practices to Theo, *when they already know she is a yoga teacher.*

What Theo is actually doing is napping, reducing stress, swimming, and taking her meds. She also decided to take a break from regular *āsana* practice for at least a year. She made this decision on the basis that if a 20-year yoga practice hasn't protected her connective tissues from damage, perhaps she should do something else for a bit.

During one of her first teacher trainings, Harriet was told that her tight hamstrings were caused by her inability to let go of the past. At the same time, her training and early period of teaching significantly delayed Harriet's recovery from disordered eating. Praised and encouraged for the shape (and shapes made) of her body, practising and teaching yoga undermined the progress she had made in therapy the two years prior. Now, Harriet is managing a variety of injuries likely to have been caused by an approach to *āsana* that was forged in the crucible of performative visual aesthetics, catalysed by a hypermobility condition that was only recognized after several years of teaching.

Like Theo, many people have suggested a variety of practices or postures to Harriet, but she suspects that backbends aren't going to cure her hamstring tendinopathy. These days, Harriet spends much more time on her feet and lifting baking trays than she does performing *caturaṅga*s and bow poses.

It is a rare yoga teacher trainer who will say this but: maybe yoga isn't the answer to everything? We know that yoga is much more than *āsana*, but maybe even meditation will not end racism, *yoga nidrā* won't cure disease, and *prāṇāyāma* won't stop climate change. Perhaps we could be better yoga teachers if we shared this fact with our students.

A FEW FINAL THOUGHTS

In the final analysis, perhaps we can usefully consider this book as a group intervention into the teaching of yoga. Like most therapeutic interventions, this one comes from a place of both love and frustration, by people who know contemporary yoga teaching intimately. We fell in love with the practice, the spaces, and the students of yoga, just as you probably did.

This book is also born in a time of global uncertainty and tension in seemingly every area of life. Perhaps every generation thinks that the issues that face it are unprecedented. But from climate change to the pandemic, from failing social systems to international conflicts, it's surprising, if not alarming, how often practices such as yoga are expected to paper over the cracks. State health systems, education providers, charities, and tech entrepreneurs prescribe this ancient and modern, Indian and cosmopolitan, powerful yet gentle, and above all ill-defined practice that everyone recognizes by the universal image of a slim white woman sitting cross-legged on the floor. They prescribe it for weight loss in the expectation that this will somehow end poverty. They prescribe it for post-traumatic stress disorder (PTSD) as a panacea for the pathologization of distress in health systems. They prescribe it to students who cannot cope with high-pressure education systems, as a way to calm prisoners caught in the carceral state, and to make underpaid workers more productive and flexible.

What everyone knows about yoga is that it is an oasis of calm, of presence, even of joy, against the vagaries of a stressful life. It releases pain and gives hope. It allows for reconciliation. We don't know if any practice alone can heal us, or the relationship we have with the world. There are certainly better ways to work for justice. But if everyone knows this about yoga, perhaps the practice can become a place where we meet to figure out how to make healing happen.

Endnotes

Introduction

1 Etienne Wenger-Trayner and Beverly Wenger-Trayner, 'Introduction to communities of practice', Wenger-Trayner, June 2015, https://wenger-trayner.com/introduction-to-communities-of-practice.

2 George Brosi, 'The beloved community: A conversation with bell hooks', *Appalachian Heritage*, 40, no. 4 (2012), 76–86.

3 Theodora Wildcroft, *Post-Lineage Yoga: From Guru to #MeToo* (Sheffield: Equinox Publishing, 2020).

4 Elizabeth De Michelis, 'A preliminary survey of modern yoga studies', *Asian Medicine*, 3 (2007), 1–19.

5 Wildcroft, *Post-Lineage Yoga*.

6 Christine Lavrence and Kristin Lozanski, '"This is not your practice life": Lululemon and the neoliberal governance of self', *Canadian Review of Sociology/Revue canadienne de sociologie*, 51 (2014), 76–94 (p. 77).

   Beatrix Hauser, 'Introduction: Transcultural Yoga(s). Analyzing a Traveling Subject', in Beatrix Hauser (ed.), *Yoga Traveling: Bodily Practice in Transcultural Perspective*, pp. 1–34 (Springer International Publishing: New York, 2013) (p. 6).

7 Hermina Drah, '34 life-altering yoga statistics & facts for a balanced 2023', MedAlertHelp.org, 2023, https://medalerthelp.org/blog/yoga-statistics.

8 Abby McCain, '25 + interesting yoga industry statistics [2023]: Yoga trends + revenue', Zippia, 20 June 2023, www.zippia.com/advice/yoga-industry-statistics.

9 Statista Research Department, 'Market size of the pilates and yoga studio sector in the United States from 2012 to 2020, with a forecast until 2022', Statista, 9 December 2022, www.statista.com/statistics/1176777/pilates-and-yoga-studio-industry-market-size-us.

10 Liz Edwards, 'Yoga Statistics', Finder UK, 23 March 2021, www.finder.com/uk/yoga-statistics.

11 Arthur Zuckerman, 'Significant yoga statistics: 2020/2021 Benefits, facts & trends', CompareCamp, 6 September 2022, https://comparecamp.com/yoga-statistics.

12 Crystal L. Park, Tosca Braun, and Tamar Siegel, 'Who practices yoga? A systematic review of demographic, health-related, and psychosocial factors associated with yoga practice', *Journal of Behavioural Medicine*, 38 (2015), 460–471 (p. 460).

13 *Yoga with Adriene* [YouTube channel], www.youtube.com/user/yogawithadriene.

14 Yoga Alliance, '2016 yoga in America study conducted by *Yoga Journal* & Yoga Alliance', Yoga Alliance, 13 January 2016, www.yogaalliance.org/2016yogainamericastudy.

15 Robert Booth, 'UK's first yoga union fights for fairer share of £900m-a-year industry', *The Guardian*, 4 February 2021, www.theguardian.com/lifeandstyle/2021/feb/04/uks-first-yoga-union-fights-for-fairer-share-of-900m-a-year-industry.

16 Michelle Goldberg, 'The brutal economics of being a yoga teacher', The Cut, 8 October 2015, http://nymag.com/thecut/2015/10/brutal-economics-of-being-a-yoga-teacher.html.

Melanie Klein, 'This is what a yogi looks like', Yoga and Body Image Coalition, 1 December 2014, http://ybicoalition.com/this-is-what-a-yogi-looks-like.

James Mallinson and Mark Singleton, *Roots of Yoga* (Penguin Books: London, 2017).

17 Theodora Wildcroft, 'Post-lineage yoga: Adventures in social media engagement', *Journal of the British Association for the Study of Religion (JBASR)*, 21 (2020), 92–113.

18 Carol Horton and Roseanne Harvey, *21st Century Yoga: Culture, Politics, and Practice* (Berkeley, CA: On Demand Publishing, LLC-Create Space, 2012) (p. 181.)

19 Tema Okun, 'Sense of Urgency', White Supremacy Culture, 2022, www.whitesupremacyculture.info/urgency.html.

20 Audre Lorde, 'The uses of anger', *Women's Studies Quarterly* 9, no. 3 (1981) (p. 9), https://academicworks.cuny.edu/cgi/viewcontent.cgi?article=1654&context=wsq.

21 Ibid.

Chapter 2

1 Mary Oliver, 'The Journey', in *Dream Work* (New York: Atlantic Monthly Press, 1986) (p. 114).

2 Mary Oliver, 'Wild Geese', in *Dream Work* (New York: Atlantic Monthly Press, 1986) (p. 110).

3 Octavio Paz, *In Light of India*, trans. Eliot Weinberger (Calcutta: 1998).

Chapter 3

1 Harriet McAtee and Amelia Wood, 'Kate Bush, power dynamics and a person-centred approach with Amelia Wood' [podcast audio], Nourish Yoga Training, *In Our Experience with Nourish Yoga Training*, 15 February 2022, https://nourishyogatraining.com/11-kate-bush-power-dynamics-and-a-person-centred-approach-with-amelia-wood.

2 Harriet McAtee and Sheena Sood, 'Yoga's liberatory potential and how we can access it with Sheena Sood' [podcast audio], Nourish Yoga Training, In Our Experience with Nourish Yoga Training, 1 March 2022, https://nourishyogatraining.com/13-yogas-liberatory-potential-and-how-we-can-access-it-with-sheena-sood.

3 Jivana Heyman, *Accessible Yoga: Poses and Practices for Every Body* (Boulder, CO: Shambala Publications, 2019) (p. 7).

4 Julia Bell, *Radical Attention* (London: Peninsula Press, 2020).

Chapter 4

1   Although *Roots of Yoga* is nominally the work of James Mallinson and Mark Singleton, it is important to note that it heavily relies on the research work of other scholars in the fields of Indology and Yoga Studies due to its enormous scope. It is a good example of the fact that the advancement of research is never a work of an inspired individual but always the whole community.

2   Renée J. Martin and Dawn M. Van Gunten, 'Reflected identities: Applying positionality and multicultural social reconstructionism in teacher education', *Journal of Teacher Education*, 53, no. 1 (2002), 44–54 (p. 46).

3   Theo Wildcroft, 'In person' (blog post) Wild Yoga, 31 January 2022, www.wildyoga. co.uk/2022/01/in-person.

4   A good, general introduction to the alternative history of India which gives voices to the unrepresented groups is the work of Wendy Doniger, in particular her book *The Hindus: An Alternative History* (Oxford: Oxford University Press, 2010). I often recommend it as an accessible work on Indian history for those who want to deepen their education beyond the history of yoga.

5   Patañjali's *Yoga Sūtra* is an obvious choice here as there are manifold translations in multiple languages, some with the commentary, some without. There are, however, other possibilities; be creative!

6   This is a term first coined by the famous French anthropologist Claude Lévi-Strauss in the 1950s. According to Lévi-Strauss, a 'floating signifier' is a word or a non-linguistic sign which has so many meanings, often ambiguous or contradictory, that it becomes essentially empty of a specific meaning. It becomes a vehicle apt to absorb meanings that readers/viewers/speakers ascribe to it, based on their personal experience. See Claude Lévi-Strauss, *Introduction to the Work of Marcel Mauss*, trans. Felicity Baker (London: Routledge & Kegan Paul, 1987) (pp. 63–64).

7   Recommended sources:

Karl Baier, Philipp André Maas, and Karin Preisendanz, *Yoga in Transformation* (Göttingen: V&R unipress, 2018), https://library.oapen.org/handle/20.500.12657/28215.

James Mallinson, and Mark Singleton, *Roots of Yoga* (London: Penguin Books, 2017).

Suzanne Newcombe and Karen O'Brien-Kop, *Routledge Handbook of Yoga and Meditation Studies* (Abingdon: Routledge, 2020).

Mark Singleton, *Yoga Body: The Origins of Modern Posture Practice* (New York: Oxford University Press, 2010).

Yogic Studies, Interview with Accessible Yoga Part 4: Modern misconceptions about early yoga (Interview with Seth Powell), 10 December 2018 www.yogicstudies.com/ blog/interview-with-accessible-yoga-part-4-modern-misconceptions-about-early-yoga.

8   Recommended sources:

Mallinson and Singleton, *Roots of Yoga*.

Seth Powell and Philipp André Maas, 'The Pātañjalayogaśāstra and its textual history' [podcast audio], Yogic Studies, *The Yogic Studies Podcast*, 4 September 2020, https:// podcast.yogicstudies.com/1046752/5282650-11-philipp-maas-the-patanjalayogasastra-and-its-textual-history.

David Gordon White, *The Yoga Sutra of Patanjali: A Biography*, Lives of Great Religious Books (Princeton, NJ: Princeton University Press, 2014).

9 Recommended sources:

James Mallinson, 'Kālavañcana in the Konkan: How a Vajrayāna Haṭhayoga tradition cheated Buddhism's death in India', *Religions (Basel, Switzerland)* 10, no. 4 (2019), 273.

Debra Diamond, *Yoga: The Art of Transformation* (Washington, DC: Arthur Sackler Gallery, 2013).

Carl W. Ernst (trans.), 'Chapter 4 of the Bahr al-hayat, by Muhammad Ghawth Gwaliyari', National Museum of Asian Art, 2013, https://asia.si.edu/essays/ocean-of-life.

Noémie Verdon, 'The Arabic Pātañjalayogaśāstra', The Luminescent, 2019, https://www.theluminescent.org/2019/10/the-arabic-patanjalayogasastra.html.

10 This is a topic which is rarely touched upon in scholarship. Therefore, I cannot recommend many sources for this, apart from this article, which touches this topic briefly: Knut A. Jacobsen, 'Yoga Powers in a Contemporary Sāṃkhya-Yoga Tradition', in Knut A. Jacobsen (ed.), *Yoga Powers: Extraordinary Capacities Attained through Meditation and Concentration* (Leiden: Brill, 2012)(pp. 459–478).

11 Recommended sources:

James Mallinson, 'Haṭha Yoga' (section Practitioners), *Brill's Encyclopedia of Hinduism Online*, vol. 3 (2011), www.academia.edu/1317005/Ha%E1%B9%ADha_Yoga_-_entry_in_Vol._3_of_the_Brill_Encyclopedia_of_Hinduism.

Mark Singleton and Ellen Goldberg (eds), *Gurus of Modern Yoga* (New York: Oxford University Press, 2013).

Theodora Wildcroft, *Post-Lineage Yoga: From Guru to #MeToo* (Sheffield: Equinox Publishing, 2020).

Chapter 6

1 Yoga Alliance, *2016 Yoga in America Study Conducted by Yoga Journal and Yoga Alliance Reveals Growth and Benefits of the Practice*, 2016, https://www.yogaalliance.org/Portals/0/YIAS%20Press%20Release%20with%20YA%20contact%20info.pdf.

2 B. S. Baum, K. Hooker, O. Vital, V. Rinsem, M. Rankin, and J. Coombs, 'Varying alignment affects lower extremity joint and limb loading during yoga's triangle (trikonasana) pose', *Journal of Bodywork and Movement Therapies* (2022), doi: 10.1016/j.jbmt.2022.02.008.

3 Y. Wu, Q. Lin, M. Yang, J. Lin et al., 'A computer vision-based yoga pose grading approach using contrastive skeleton feature representations', *Healthcare*, 10, (2021), 36.

4 S. J. Wilcox, R. Hager, B. Lockhart, and M. K. Seeley, 'Ground reaction forces generated by twenty-eight hatha yoga postures', *International Journal of Exercise Science*, 5 (2012), 114–126.

5 H. Cramer, L. Ward, R. Saper, D. Fishbein, G. Dobos, and R. Lauche, 'The safety of yoga: A systematic review and meta-analysis of randomized controlled trials', *American Journal of Epidemiology*, 182 (2015), 281–293.

6 J. T. Chandler and M. H. Stone, 'The squat exercise in athletic conditioning: A review of the literature', *National Strength and Conditioning Association Journal*, 3, no. 5 (1991), 51–60.

7 H. Cramer et al., 'The safety of yoga'.

8   D. Yosifon and P. N. Stearns, 'The rise and fall of American posture', *American Historical Review*, 103, no. 4 (1998), 1057–1095.

9   D. G. Behm, *The Science and Physiology of Flexibility and Stretching: Implications and Applications in Sport Performance and Health* (1st edn) (Abingdon: Routledge, 2018).

10   ACSM 5 components of fitness: strength, endurance, flexibility, neuromotor fitness, body mass index. American College of Sports Medicine, *ACSM's Health-Related Physical Fitness Assessment Manual* (5th edn) (Philadelphia, PA: Lippincott Williams and Wilkins, 2017), www.acsm.org/docs/default-source/publications-files/hrpfam5_table-8-9-updated.pdf?sfvrsn=e82139fc_4.

11   H. Chaabene, D. G. Behm, Y. Negra, and U. Granacher, 'Acute effects of static stretching on muscle strength and power: An attempt to clarify previous caveats', *Frontiers in Physiology*, 10 (2019), 1468.

12   S. S. Y. Yu, M.-Y. Wang, S. Samarawickrame, R. Hashish et al., 'The physical demands of the tree (vriksasana) and one-leg balance (utthita hasta padagusthasana) poses performed by seniors: A biomechanical examination', *Evidence-Based Complementary Alternative Medicine* (2012), doi: 10.1155/2012/971896.

13   Cramer, 'Safety of yoga'.

14   Yosifon and Sterns, 'Rise and fall'.

15   D. G. Behm, A. J. Blazevich, A. D. Kay, and M. McHugh, 'Acute effects of muscle stretching on physical performance, range of motion, and injury incidence in healthy active individuals: A systematic review', *Applied Physiology, Nutrition, and Metabolism*, 41 (2015), 1–11.

16   Chaabene, 'Acute Effects'.

17   V. Korakakis, K. O'Sullivan, P. B. O'Sullivan, V. Evagelinou, et al., 'Physiotherapist perceptions of optimal sitting and standing posture', *Musculoskeletal Science and Practice*, 39 (2019), 24–31.

Chapter 7

1   Paul Rowe, Adam Koller, and Sandeep Sharma, 'Physiology, bone remodeling', StatPearls, 17 March 2023, www.ncbi.nlm.nih.gov/books/NBK499863.

2   H. G. Davis, *Conservative Surgery* (New York: Appleton, 1867).

Chapter 8

1   *Sthira-sukha-āsanam* – E. F. Bryant (trans.), *The Yoga Sūtra of Patañjali* (2.46) (New York: North Point Press, 2009) (p. 283).

2   Linda Hartley, *Somatic Psychology* (London: Wiley, 2004) (p. 153).

3   Linda Hartley, *Wisdom of the Body Moving* (Berkeley, CA: North Atlantic Books, 1995) (p. 124).

4   A question first formulated in a 1995 paper entitled *Facing Up To The Problem of Consciousness* (http://consc.net/papers/facing.pdf) by David Chalmers, now Professor of Philosophy and Neuroscience at the University of New York and co-director of NYU Center for Mind, Brain, and Consciousness.

5   Maurice Merleau-Ponty, 'The Visible and the Unvisible' (1968), trans. Michael B. Smith, in *The Merleau Ponty Aesthetics Reader* (Chicago: Northwestern University Press, 1993) (p. 125).

6   *atha yogānuśāsanam* – Bryant, *Yoga Sūtra of Patañjali* (1.1) (p. 4).

7   *yogaścittavṛttinirodhaḥ* – Bryant, *Yoga Sūtra of Patañjali* (1.2) (p. 4).

8   Elizabeth De Michelis, 'A preliminary survey of modern yoga studies', *Asian Medicine* 3 (2007), 1–19.

9   See Bryant, *Yoga Sūtra of Patañjali*, xxv–xxx.

10 *pratyakṣānumānāgamāḥ pramāṇāni* – Bryant, *Yoga Sutra of Patañjali* (1.7) (p. 32).

11 See Bryant, *Yoga Sūtra of Patañjali*, 9.

12 Bryant, *Yoga Sūtra of Patañjali* (2.54–2.55, 3.1–2) (pp. 297–310).

13 See Patrizia Pallaro (ed.), *Authentic Movement* (London: Jessica Kingsley Publishers, 1999).

14 Bonnie Bainbridge Cohen, *Sensing, Feeling, and Action* (3rd edn) (Middletown, CT: Wesleyan University Press, 2008) (p. 157).

15 'Man muss Geduld haben mit dem ungelösten im Herzen, und versuchen, die Fragen selber lieb zu haben, wie verschlossene Stuben, und wie Bücher, die in einer sehr fremden Sprache eschrieben sind. Es handelt sich darum, alles zu leben. Wenn man die Fragen lebt, lebt man vielleicht allmählich, ohne es zu merken, eines fremden Tages in die Antworten hinein': Rainier Maria Rilke, *Letters to a Young Poet*, trans. Stephen Mitchell (New York: Random House, 1984) (p. 34).

Chapter 9

1   Judith Herman, *Trauma and Recovery: The Aftermath of Violence – from Domestic Abuse to Political Terror* (New York: Basic Books, 1992) (p. 7).

2   Ibid.

3   Caroline Alexander, 'The shock of war', *Smithsonian Magazine*, 1 September 2010, www.smithsonianmag.com/history/the-shock-of-war-55376701.

4   E. Jones and S. Wessely, *Shell Shock to PTSD: Military Psychiatry from 1900 to the Gulf War* (Abingdon: Taylor & Francis Group, 2006) (p. 19).

5   Herman, *Trauma and Recovery*, 21.

6   Ibid., 20.

7   Ibid., 10.

8   Ibid., 11.

9   Ibid., 12.

10 Ibid., 13–14.

11 Jones & Wessely, *Shell Shock to PTSD*, 111.

12 Ibid., 148.

13 Bessel Van der Kolk, *The Body Keeps the Score: Mind, Brain and Body in the Transformation of Trauma* (London: Penguin Random House, 2014) (p. 1).

14 Van der Kolk, *Body Keeps the Score*, 359–361.

15 Herman, *Trauma and Recovery*, 8.

16 Lisa Oakley and Kathryn Kinmond, *Breaking the Silence on Spiritual Abuse* (Basingstoke: Palgrave Macmillan, 2013) (pp. 21–22).

17 Royal Commission into Institutional Responses to Child Sexual Abuse, 'Case Study No. 21: Satyananda Yoga Ashram', www.childabuseroyalcommission.gov.au/case-studies/case-study-21-satyananda-yoga-ashram.

18 Jack Healy, 'Schism emerges in bikram yoga empire amid rape claims', *New York Times*, 23 February 2015, www.nytimes.com/2015/02/24/us/cracks-show-in-bikram-yoga-empire-amid-claims-of-rape-and-assault.html.

19 Andrea Jain, *Peace Love Yoga: The Politics of Global Spirituality* (Oxford: Oxford University Press, 2020) (p. 102).

20 Matthew Remski, *Practice and All Is Coming: Abuse, Cult Dynamics, and Healing in Yoga and Beyond* (Rangiora, New Zealand: Embodied Wisdom Publishing Ltd, 2019).

21 Philip Deslippe, 'From Maharaj to Mahan Tantric: The construction of Yogi Bhajan's Kundalini Yoga', *Sikh Formations*, 8 (2012), 369–387.

Chapter 10

1   'Trauma and Yoga Series Part 1: Why Agency Is Everything in Trauma-Informed Spaces', Nourish Yoga Training, 10 March 2022, https://nourishyogatraining.com/trauma-and-yoga-series-part-1-why-agency-is-everything-in-trauma-informed-spaces-2.

    'Trauma and Yoga Series Part 2: What You Need to Know about Trauma-Informed Teacher Trainings', Nourish Yoga Training, 11 April 2022, https://nourishyogatraining.com/trauma-and-yoga-series-part-1-why-agency-is-everything-in-trauma-informed-spaces.

2   James W. Moore, 'What is the sense of agency and why does it matter?' *Frontiers in Psychology*, 7 (2016), 1272.

3   Chris C. Streeter, Patricia L. Gerbarg, et al., 'Treatment of major depressive disorder with Iyengar yoga and coherent breathing: A randomized controlled dosing study', *Journal of Alternative and Complementary Medicine*, 23, no. 3 (2017), 201–207.

Chapter 12

1   Sheena Sood, 'Towards a critical embodiment of decolonizing yoga', *Race and Yoga*, http://dx.doi.org/10.5070/R351049160.

2   Edward W. Said, *Orientalism* (London: Penguin, 2021) (p. 3).

3   Ibid., 25.

4   Personal conversation with Sheena Sood.

5   Ezra Klein, Joe Posner, and Chad Mumm (Producers), 'Mindfulness', season 1, episode 4 of *The Mind, Explained*, Netflix (Vox Media, 2019), www.netflix.com/gb/title/81098586.

6   Ibid.

7   'Yogis for Palestine: A call to action in solidarity with Palestine', www.yogis4palestine.com.

Chapter 13

1   Paulo Freire, *Pedagogy of the Oppressed* (Penguin: London, 1996) (p. 27).

2   bell hooks, *Teaching to Transgress: Education as the Practice of Freedom* (New York: Routledge, 1996).

3   Emma Dabiri, *What White People Can Do Next: From Allyship to Coalition* (London: Penguin Books, 2021).

4   Jason Okundaye, 'Author Emma Dabiri on what white people can do right now', *British Vogue*, 14 April 2021, www.vogue.co.uk/arts-and-lifestyle/article/emma-dabiri-what-white-people-can-do-next.

5   Freire, *Pedagogy of the Oppressed*, 27.

6   Karl Marx and Friedrich Engels, *The Communist Manifesto*.

7   Thomas Sankara, 'Thomas Sankara on the power of solidarity', *Tribune*, 15 October 2021, https://tribunemag.co.uk/2021/10/thomas-sankara-on-the-power-of-solidarity.

8   Harriet McAtee, 19. Performance or Practice and the Nature of Rest with Beverley Nolan, Nourish Yoga Training (n.d.), https://nourishyogatraining.com/19-performance-or-practice-and-the-nature-of-rest-with-beverley-nolan.

Chapter 15

1   Oxford University Press, 'Capitalism', 2023, Oxford Learners Dictionaries, www.oxfordlearnersdictionaries.com/definition/american_english/capitalism.

2   Yoga Teachers Union, *The Money Side of Teaching: Earnings & Salaries in the UK*, 2019, https://drive.google.com/file/d/1oCLi4PPXv-xnWr--7HColjwaZpv-vYHv/view.

3   Yoga Teachers Union, 2020 Survey Overview, 2020, https://drive.google.com/file/d/1L b5JoCXT1gIqCs6LAywS7dTRD4yQKiq6/view.

4   Donna Farhi, *Teaching Yoga: Exploring the Teacher–Student Relationship* (Berkeley, CA: Rodmell, 2006) (p. 111).

5   Email exchange with Adam Ohringer, employment law barrister.

6   Sarah Jaffe, *Work Won't Love You Back: How Devotion to Our Jobs Keeps Us Exploited, Exhausted and Alone* (London: C. Hurst & Co, 2022) (p. 13).

7   Diemut Bubeck, *Care, Gender and Justice* (Oxford: Clarendon Press, 1995) (p. 9).

8   Yoga Teachers Union, *Money Side of Teaching*.

9   Chiara Bottici, *Anarchafeminism* (London: Bloomsbury Academic, 2022).

10 Maria Mies, *Patriarchy and Accumulation on a World Scale: Women in the International Division of Labour* (London: Zed Books, 2001).

11 Bottici, *Anarchafeminism*, 17.

12 Yoga Teachers Union, *Money Side of Teaching*.

13 Amber Husain, *Replace Me* (London: Peninsula Press, 2021) (p. 35).

14 *Uber BV and Others (Appellants) v Aslam and Others (Respondents)*, 2021, UKSC 5, www.supremecourt.uk/cases/docs/uksc-2019-0029-judgment.pdf.

15 Royal Society of Arts, Gig economy chart (n.d.), www.thersa.org/globalassets/images/infographics/rsa-gig-economy-chart.pdf.

16 Emily Scurrah, Alice Martin, Aidan Harper, and Rachel Laurence, *Beyond the Gig Economy: Empowering the Self-Employed Workforce*, New Economics Foundation, 2020, https://neweconomics.org/uploads/files/NEF_Empowering-self-employed-workforce.pdf.

17 Ibid., 4.

18 Bubeck, *Care, Gender and Justice*, 7.

19 Jaffe, *Work Won't Love You Back*, 8.

Chapter 16

1   Brigid Delaney, 'The yoga industry is booming – but does it make you a better person?' *The Guardian*, 17 September 2017, www.theguardian.com/lifeandstyle/2017/sep/17/yoga-better-person-lifestyle-exercise.

2   According to a mapping exercise carried out by the author for the IWGB Yoga Teachers Union.

3   In 2022, there were over 700 members of the Yoga Teachers Brighton Facebook group alone.

4   Sadly a video recording of the event was not organized.

5   Tom Walker, 'United Fitness Brands snaps up Triyoga', Leisure Opportunities, 4 January 2022, www.leisureopportunities.co.uk/news/United-Fitness-Brands-adds-Triyoga-to-portfolio-of-boutique-operators-Kobox-Boom-Cycle-Barrecore-Joe-Cohen-Jonathan-Sattin/348974.

6   Insolvency Intel, Yoga London Ltd: Appointment of Liquidators, 2022, https://insolvencyintel.co.uk/yoga-london-ltd.

7   Matt McGrath, 'Climate change: IPCC report warns of "irreversible" impacts of global warming', *BBC News*, 28 February 2022, https://www.bbc.co.uk/news/science-environment-60525591.

Chapter 17

1   Jivana Heyman, *Accessible Yoga: Poses and Practices for Every Body* (Boulder, CO: Shambhala, 2019). Jivana Heyman, *Yoga Revolution: Building a Practice of Courage and Compassion* (Boulder, CO: Shambhala, 2021).

2   Juan Mascaró (trans.), *The Upanishads* (Harmondsworth: Penguin, 1965) (p. 120).

3   Sonya Renee Taylor, *The Body Is Not an Apology* (Oakland, CA: Berrett-Koehler Publishers, 2021).

4   Jaganath Carrera, *Inside the Yoga Sutras: A Comprehensive Sourcebook for the Study and Practice of Patanjali's Yoga Sutras* (Buckingham, VA: Integral Yoga Publications, 2006), 42–52.

5   Satchidananda, *The Living Gita: The Complete Bhagavad Gita: A Commentary for Modern Readers* (Yogaville, VA: Integral Yoga Publications, 1988) (p. 91).

Conclusion

1   https://judemills.com/podcast.

Index